Competency
Check-Off Guides

Building Confidence Through
Core Competency Checklists

Competency Check-Off Guides

Building Confidence Through
Core Competency Checklists

KRIS A. HARDY, AS, CMA, RHE, CDF

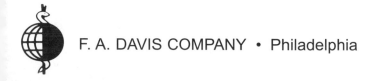

F. A. DAVIS COMPANY • Philadelphia

F. A. Davis Company
1915 Arch Street
Philadelphia, PA 19103
www.fadavis.com

Printed in the United States of America

Last digit indicates print number: 10 9 8 7 6 5 4 3 2 1

Acquisitions Editor: Andy McPhee
Manager, Content Development: Deborah Thorp
Developmental Editor: Melissa Reed
Art and Design Manager: Carolyn O'Brien

As new scientific information becomes available through basic and clinical research, recommended treatments and drug therapies undergo changes. The author(s) and publisher have done everything possible to make this book accurate, up to date, and in accord with accepted standards at the time of publication. The author(s), editors, and publisher are not responsible for errors or omissions or for consequences from application of the book, and make no warranty, expressed or implied, in regard to the contents of the book. Any practice described in this book should be applied by the reader in accordance with professional standards of care used in regard to the unique circumstances that may apply in each situation. The reader is advised always to check product information (package inserts) for changes and new information regarding dose and contraindications before administering any drug. Caution is especially urged when using new or infrequently ordered drugs.

ISBN 0-8036-1468-3

Dedication

I took great pleasure in writing and creating these competency check-off tools, and I take even greater pleasure in sharing these tools with you. Everyone knows that trying to adequately satisfy the standards in competency format is no easy feat. After my first site visit and several citations to competency check-off, I decided I was going to build a tool that was easy and formatted to the standards that came in one simple complete package and could be used with any core text.

I dedicate this competency check-off manual to all the faculty and program directors/coordinators that are up for reaccreditation or are applying for accreditation for the first time by either CAAHEP or ABHES. May this manual make your job easier and instill a quality sense of direction and instruction for your students.

Author Acknowledgments

First, I must thank my faithful and devoted husband, Patrick Hardy, who has stood by my every endeavor both personally and professionally. Without his constant support, encouragement, and involvement, this publication would not be possible. His willingness to allow me to grow as a professional and set his own needs aside is to be commended and never forgotten. He has truly been the man of my dreams and has helped me to achieve my goals.

Without the love and encouragement from my mother and father, Phyllis and Larry Tilford, and my brothers, Bryan and Lance Tilford, I would not be where I am today. I am forever grateful in their belief in my ability to achieve even when I thought it was not possible.

Special thanks to my dear friends and colleagues, Patricia Rock, LPN, Deborah Verillo, BSN, and Darcy Roy, CMA, CPC, for their years of input in helping to define quality competency. I am privileged to know and love such caring, nurturing, and excellent health care practitioners and educators.

Thanks to Michelle Carfagna, RMA, who assisted with the competency organization.

I would like to thank my employer, Brevard Community College, who has provided me with the opportunity to grow in many different directions both personally and professionally. They have instilled a sense of pride about how and what I teach.

Lastly, I give thanks to F. A. Davis. It only seems fitting that they publish my first works. I have in my possession, passed down from family generations, some very early publications by F. A. Davis called *Sajous's Analytical Cyclopaedia of Practical Medicine*, Volumes I–IV, published in 1902, which my great, great, grandfather, Franklin Pierce Tilford, used as he practiced medicine. It contains many notes scribbled about patients owing him chickens in return for services and his completion notes from medical school in 1879. I can only imagine this was one of his first sets of medical publications. While we all learn and strive through different generations and instruction, F. A. Davis had faith in me just as my great, great, grandfather had faith in the knowledge and instruction he received from these early publications. Thank you F. A. Davis for keeping medicine on the front line and extending your publications for and from so many generations.

KRIS A. HARDY, AS, CMA, RHE, CDF
Program Director/Medical Assistant Program
Brevard Community College, Cocoa, FL

Reviewers

CAROLE BERUBE, MA, MSN, BSN, RN
Professor Emerita, Medical Assisting Program
Health Sciences Department
Bristol Community College
Fall River, MA

URSULA E. COLE, MAED, BAED, CMA, CCS-P, RHE
Chairperson, Medical Curriculum
Indiana Business College
Terre Haute, IN

MARY ANNE CRANDALL, RN, BS, MS
Instructor, Extended Campus Programs
Southern Oregon University
Ashland, OR

JEANNE GRIFFITH, BS
Director of Training
OIC Training Academy
Barracksville, WV

TONYA HALLOCK, MA
Librarian and Director, Medical Assisting Program
Concorde Career Institute
Garden Grove, CA

BRENDA HARTSON, MSM, BSM, CMA
Manager, Medical Assisting Program
Colorado Technical University
Sioux Falls, SD

JOYCE MINTON, BS, CMA, RMA
Director, Medical Assisting Program
Health Sciences Department
Wilkes Community College
Wilkesboro, NC

ONA SCHULZ, CMA
Instructor and Coordinator, Medical Assisting
  Program
Allied Health Department
Lake Washington Technical College
Kirkland, WA

BARBARA TIETSORT, MED
Associate Professor, Office Information Technology
  and Medical Assisting
University of Cincinnati
Cincinnati, OH

MARILYN TURNER, RN, CMA
Director, Medical Assisting Program
Chair, Health Sciences Department
Ogeechee Technical College
Statesboro, GA

BENNITA VAUGHANS, RN, BSN
Instructor and Coordinator, Medical Assisting
  Program
H. Councill Trenholm State Technical College
Montgomery, AL

Contents

Appendix

Index, 256

Preface

Who Is It for? Why Is It Important?

Competency Check-Off Guides: Building Confidence Through Core Competency Checklists is designed for students enrolled in medical assistant programs where competency and performance-based check-off are mandatory by Accrediting Bureau of Health Education Schools (ABHES) or Commission on Accreditation of Allied Health Education Programs (CAAHEP). The information and practicums presented are designed to enhance any allied health career program where step-by-step task instruction for administrative or clinical procedures is required.
Hands-on technical skills remain and will always be a high priority. Learning these skills is essential to the success of today's health care workers and the patients that are served.

Students, who become health care employees, must understand the need to perform in a professional, ethical, legal, and competent manner. These competencies will help develop and strengthen skills while building confidence.
This competency check-off manual was designed to introduce the student to real-life scenarios through interaction with their fellow classmates, laboratory equipment and supplies, and classroom theory by performing administrative, clinical, and general competencies that will help build confidence for actual task performance.
The competencies are linked to real standards to ensure that all programs, whether seeking accreditation or not, are providing opportunities for students to achieve excellence in entry-level skills.

These competencies are also designed with the instructor/program director-coordinator in mind and will help programs meet the standards for competency-based format. Built into one complete package, the task of gathering and matching competencies to standards has been done for you.

What Is Covered in This Manual?

Text Organization
The manual begins with the medical office **Database** where students will find information about the practice and patients. Students will refer to the Database periodically for practice information, which will help them to successfully complete the competencies in a real-world fashion. Information not found in the Database has been built into the actual competency as well as all the forms needed to complete the task with accuracy.

The manual is then divided into two main sections: **Administrative/General** and **Clinical/General Competencies**. Each section contains the competency standards set forth by CAAHEP and ABHES, linked together in a performance based, step-by-step learning approach for the student.

Key Features
Throughout all of the competencies, Dr. Wright has provided reminders called "Make a Difference" that coincide with the practice philosophy and initiate a quality commitment to the patients and the practice. The **Make a Difference** boxes will provide you with reminders from your theory-based lecture, which will help with retention and provide helpful tips for the future.

Standard Precautions have been addressed in every clinical competency. The clinical components are in strict alignment with health-care standards in hopes that students will continue to practice standards once they are a graduate and a credentialed health care employee.

In many of the step-by-step tasks, **Dr. Wright** has provided useful tips to explain the purpose of why the student is performing the task that way and how important it is to follow standards and protocol and/or how to achieve this task step with quality assurance.

In many of the competencies, **Smart Thinking** will also aid the student with questions that will assist in retention skills of important terms and in critically thinking areas. Answers to the questions are found in the back of the manual. The majority of the competencies require **Documentation** in charting form or actual task performance to provide a repetitious learning experience. This will help ensure proficiency of mastering the skill of charting and documentation.

Students should have an understanding of the nature of the profession that they have chosen and what entry-level skills they are expected to learn. The **Entry-Level Theory and Competency** by both CAAHEP and ABHES has been provided in this manual to assist students in understanding the importance of accredited programs and the standards by which they are taught. The student must recognize the reason behind what they are learning to become competent health care workers. Accredited programs must supply this information to the student at the beginning of the program to meet the standards. This task has also been done for you.

Performance Criteria/Evaluation Accumulation is included and will allow the instructor to carry forward the achievements of each competency onto one grading form. This will assist in making the final task of adding points or figuring grades easier. This also allows students to identify each performance objective along with its major category and provides students with a better understanding of the standard and their progress.

To the Student

Students should read the Specific Task at the beginning of each competency and then review each task step. Pay special attention to the Make a Difference boxes, Standard Precautions, and the Equipment/Supplies needed because these will also help lead you to a successful check-off. Practice and role-play as much as you can to enhance your skill level. Many of the check-offs are designed to be performed with a classmate to enhance your confidence for the externship experience and employment.

After adequate practice, the instructor will either watch you perform and/or assign a time frame for you to complete each competency. The instructor will decide at his/her discretion how many attempts are needed to pass each competency.

Many of the competencies require documentation and/or questions (Smart Thinking) to completely satisfy the entire competency.

Your instructor will inform you which competency you will work on and when the due date for each check-off is. The instructor will inform you of any change in the task step or equipment or supplies used. The more you practice, the more you will become confident in your skill!

To the Instructor

Achievement/Grading

The faculties may choose to test the student on a pass or fail status or a grade or point value can be assigned. Simply add to your syllabus how the student will achieve each competency and its worth to complete satisfaction of the standards. Enclosed you will find a Performance Criteria Grading Form. This enables the instructor to carry forward the achievements of the student from each competency on one page for easier grade point accumulation. Although there are 5 points assigned to each competency, how you determine the achievement of each competency is completely up to you.

Allow adequate practice time for the student to help them achieve a successful check-off, guiding the student where applicable.

Some competencies may vary depending on the availability of your equipment and/or supplies. Let the student know in advance of any variations to the task steps.

Many of the competencies are linked together in a fashion that represents how they all tie together in the real world. This allows the student to understand and prepare for good time management skills. Regardless of standards/ competencies that are revised, added, or deleted, it is important that the student realize how and where these steps and tasks join one another in the real clinic/office setting.

All competencies match standard lecture format and can be used with any core text for medical assistant/ allied health instruction. This competency-based format is matched to the latest and revised standards from both CAAHEP and ABHES and covers all three components:

(1)   Specific task to be mastered
(2)   Conditions under which the student is expected to perform the task
(3)   Standard of performance for the task

PART 1
Performance Criteria

American Association of Medical Assistants (AAMA)/CAAHEP

Performance Criteria – Evaluation Accumulation

Student Name:_____

There are 65 competencies total. At 5 points each, the student can achieve up to 325 points.
Administrative/General: 31 competencies for a total of 155 points
Clinical/General: 34 competencies for a total of 170 points

Having completed each competency successfully, the student will be able to:

ADMINISTRATIVE/GENERAL

Grade/Points/Pass-Fail

LEGAL CONCEPTS

Practicum 2

_____   3. c. (2) (a)   Identify and respond to issues of confidentiality

Practicum 3

_____   3. c. (2) (b)   Perform within legal and ethical boundaries

Practicum 4

_____   3. c. (2) (f)   Demonstrate knowledge of federal and state health-care legislation and regulations

_____   *Total Points – Pass or Fail*

PATIENT INSTRUCTION

OFFICE POLICIES

Practicum 5

_____   3. c. (3) (a)   Explain general office policies

Practicum 6

_____   3. c. (3) (b)   Instruct individuals according to their needs
_____   3. c. (3) (c)   Provide instruction for health maintenance and disease prevention

Practicum 7

_____   3. c. (3) (d)   Identify community resources

_____   *Total Points – Pass or Fail*

PERFORM CLERICAL FUNCTIONS

OPERATIONAL FUNCTIONS

PROFESSIONAL COMMUNICATION

PROCESS INSURANCE CLAIMS

LEGAL CONCEPTS

PERFORM BOOKKEEPING PROCEDURES

Practicum 9

_____	3. a. (1) (a)	Schedule and manage appointments
_____	3. c. (4) (c)	Utilize computer software to maintain office systems
_____	3. c. (1) (d)	Demonstrate telephone technique

Practicum 10

_____	3. a. (1) (b)	Schedule inpatient and outpatient admissions and procedures
_____	3. a. (3) (a)	Apply managed-care policies and procedures

Practicum 11

_____	3. a. (1) (c)	Organize a patient's medical record
_____	3. a. (1) (d)	File medical records
_____	3. c. (2) (c)	Establish and maintain the medical record

Practicum 15

_____	3. a. (2) (a)	Prepare a bank deposit

Practicum 16

_____	3. a. (2) (b)	Post entries on a day sheet
_____	3. a. (2) (c)	Perform accounts receivable procedures
_____	3. a. (2) (e)	Post adjustments
_____	3. a. (2) (f)	Process credit balance
_____	3. a. (2) (g)	Process refunds
_____	3. a. (2) (h)	Post NSF checks
_____	3. a. (2) (i)	Post collection agency payments

Practicum 17

_____	3. a. (2) (d)	Perform billing and collection procedures

Practicum 18

_____	3. a. (3) (b)	Apply third-party guidelines
_____	3. c. (1) (a)	Respond to and initiate written communication

Practicum 19

_____	3. a. (3) (c)	Perform procedural coding
_____	3. a. (3) (d)	Perform diagnostic coding
_____	3. a. (3) (e)	Complete insurance claim forms

Practicum 20

_____	3. c. (4) (a)	Perform an inventory of supplies and equipment
_____	3. c. (4) (b)	Perform routine maintenance of administrative and clinical equipment

_____   ***Total Points – Pass or Fail***

CLINICAL/GENERAL

Grade/Points/Pass-Fail

FUNDAMENTAL PROCEDURES

PATIENT CARE

LEGAL CONCEPTS

PROFESSIONAL COMMUNICATION

Practicum 22

_____   3. b. (1) (a)   Perform hand washing

Practicum 23

_____   3. b. (4) (a)   Perform telephone and in-person screening

Practicum 24

_____   3. b. (4) (b)   Obtain vital signs
_____   3. c. (2) (e)   Document appropriately

Practicum 25

_____   3. b. (4) (c)   Obtain and record patient history
_____   3. c. (1) (b)   Recognize and respond to verbal communication
_____   3. c. (1) (c)   Recognize and respond to nonverbal communication

Practicum 26

_____   3. b. (4) (d)   Prepare and maintain examination and treatment areas

Practicum 27

_____   3. b. (4) (e)   Prepare patient for and assist with routine and specialty examinations
_____   3. b. (2) (e)   Instruct patients in the collection of fecal specimens

Practicum 28

_____   3. b. (4) (f)   Prepare patient for and assist with procedures, treatments, and minor office surgery
_____   3. b. (1) (b)   Wrap items for autoclaving
_____   3. b. (1) (c)   Perform sterilization techniques

Practicum 29

_____   3. b. (4) (g)   Apply pharmacology principles to prepare and administer oral and parenteral (excluding intravenous [IV]) medications

Practicum 30

_____   3. b. (4) (g)   Apply pharmacology principles to prepare and administer oral and parenteral (excluding IV) medications

Practicum 31

_____   3. b. (4) (h)   Maintain medication and immunization records

Practicum 32

_____   3. b. (4) (i)   Screen and follow up test results

_____   ***Total Points – Pass or Fail***

SPECIMEN COLLECTION

DIAGNOSTIC TESTING

LEGAL CONCEPTS

FUNDAMENTAL PROCEDURES

Practicum 33

_____	3. b. (1) (d)	Dispose of biohazardous materials
_____	3. b. (1) (e)	Practice standard precaution
_____	3. b. (2) (a)	Perform venipuncture
_____	3. c. (2) (e)	Document appropriately

_____   *Total Points – Pass or Fail*

Practicum 34

_____	3. b. (2) (b)	Perform capillary puncture
_____	3. b. (3) (c)	CLIA Waived Tests
	(iii)	Perform chemistry tests
_____	3. c. (4) (d)	Use methods of quality control

Practicum 35

_____	3. b. (2) (c)	Obtain specimens for microbiological testing
_____	3. b. (3) (c)	CLIA Waived Tests
	(v)	Perform microbiology testing

Practicum 36

_____	3. b. (2) (d)	Instruct patients in the collection of a clean-catch mid-stream urine

Practicum 37

_____	3. b. (3) (c)	CLIA Waived Tests
	(ii)	Perform hematology testing

Practicum 38

_____	3. b. (3) (c)	CLIA Waived Tests
	(iv)	Perform immunology testing

Practicum 39

_____	3. c. (4) (d)	Use methods of quality control
_____	3. b. (3) (c)	CLIA Waived Tests
	(i)	Perform urinalysis

_____   *Total Points – Pass or Fail*

Practicum 40

_____	3. b. (3) (a)	Perform electrocardiography

Practicum 41

_____	3. b. (3) (b)	Perform respiratory testing

_____   *Total Points – Pass or Fail*

PROFESSIONAL COMPONENTS

Practicum 42

_____   Provider-level cardiopulmonary resuscitation (CPR) certification and
first aid training

Achieved   Not Achieved
Date _____

Card Attached: Yes   No

The student named above:
_____   HAS achieved proficiency in the performance objectives.
_____   HAS NOT achieved proficiency in the performance objectives.

American Medical Technologists (AMT)/ABHES

Performance Objectives – Evaluation Accumulation

Student Name:_____

There are 111 competencies total. At 5 points each, the student can achieve up to 555 points.
Administrative/General: 63 competencies for a total of 315 points
Clinical/General: 48 competencies for a total of 240

Having completed each competency successfully, the student will be able to:

ADMINISTRATIVE/GENERAL

Grade/Points/Pass-Fail

PROFESSIONALISM

LEGAL CONCEPTS

COMMUNICATION

OFFICE MANAGEMENT

Practicum 1

_____	1. (f)	Adapt to change

Practicum 2

_____	1. (b)	Maintain confidentiality at all times
_____	5. (c)	Use appropriate guidelines when releasing records or information

Practicum 3

_____	1. (a)	Project a positive attitude
_____	1. (d)	Be cognizant of ethical boundaries
_____	1. (g)	Evidence a responsible attitude
_____	1. (i)	Conduct work within scope of education, training, and ability
_____	2. (p)	Professional components
_____	2. (q)	Allied health professions and credentialing
_____	5. (f)	Maintain licenses and accreditation
_____	6. (e)	Maintain liability coverage

_____   *Total Points – Pass or Fail*

LEGAL CONCEPTS

INSTRUCTION

COMMUNICATION

Practicum 4

_____	5. (e)	Dispose of controlled substances in compliance with government regulations
_____	5. (g)	Monitor legislation related to current health-care issues and practices

Practicum 5

_____	7. (a)	Orient patients to office policies and procedures

Practicum 6

_____	2. (c)	Adapt what is said to the recipient's level of comprehension
_____	2. (m)	Adaptation for individualized needs
_____	7. (b)	Instruct patients with special needs
_____	7. (c)	Teach patients methods of health promotion and disease prevention

_____   **Total Points – Pass or Fail**

ADMINISTRATIVE DUTIES

COMMUNICATION

INSTRUCTION

Practicum 7

_____	3. (f)	Locate resources and information for patients and employers
_____	7. (b)	Instruct patients with special needs

Practicum 8

_____	3. (g)	Manage physician's professional schedule and travel

Practicum 9

_____	2. (e)	Use proper telephone techniques
_____	2. (n)	Application of electronic technology
_____	3. (c)	Schedule and monitor appointments
_____	3. (d)	Apply computer concepts for office procedures

Practicum 10

_____	3. (h)	Schedule inpatient and outpatient admissions
_____	3. (u)	Apply managed care policies and procedures
_____	3. (v)	Obtain managed care referrals and precertification

Practicum 11

_____	3. (b)	Prepare and maintain medical records
_____	3. (i)	File medical records

_____   **Total Points – Pass or Fail**

LEGAL CONCEPTS:

ADMINISTRATIVE DUTIES:

FINANCIAL MANAGEMENT:

Practicum 12

_____	5. (d)	Follow established policy in initiating or terminating medical treatment

Practicum 13

_____	3. (e)	Perform medical transcriptions

Practicum 14

_____	3. (o)	Establish and maintain a petty cash fund

Practicum 15

_____	3. (a)	Perform basic secretarial skills
_____	3. (j)	Prepare a bank statement
_____	3. (k)	Reconcile a bank statement
_____	8. (e)	Maintain records for accounting and banking purposes

Practicum 16

_____	3. (l)	Post entries on a day sheet
_____	3. (n)	Prepare a check
_____	3. (p)	Post adjustments
_____	3. (q)	Process credit balance
_____	3. (r)	Process refunds
_____	3. (s)	Post NSF funds
_____	3. (t)	Post collection agency payments
_____	8. (a)	Use manual and computerized bookkeeping systems
_____	8. (d)	Manage accounts payable and receivable

_____   **Total Points – Pass or Fail**

PROFESSIONALISM

COMMUNICATION

ADMINISTRATIVE DUTIES

OFFICE MANAGEMENT

FINANCIAL MANAGEMENT

Practicum 17

_____	1. (h)	Be courteous and diplomatic
_____	2. (d)	Serve as a liaison between the physician and others
_____	3. (m)	Perform billing and collection procedures
_____	6. (f)	Exercise efficient time management

Practicum 18

_____	2. (h)	Receive, organize, prioritize, and transmit information expediently
_____	2. (o)	Fundamental writing skills
_____	8. (c)	Analyze and use current third-party guidelines for reimbursement

Practicum 19

_____	3. (w)	Perform diagnostic coding
_____	3. (x)	Complete insurance claim forms
_____	3. (y)	Use physician fee schedule
_____	8. (b)	Implement current procedural terminology and ICD-9 coding

_____   **Total Points – Pass or Fail**

OFFICE MANAGEMENT

INSTRUCTION

FINANCIAL MANAGEMENT

Practicum 20

_____	6. (a)	Maintain physical plant
_____	6. (b)	Operate and maintain facilities and equipment safely
_____	6. (c)	Inventory equipment and supplies
_____	6. (d)	Evaluate and recommend equipment and supplies for practice
_____	7. (d)	Orient and train personnel

Practicum 21

_____	8. (f)	Process employee payroll

_____   ***Total Points – Pass or Fail***

CLINICAL/GENERAL

COMMUNICATION

CLINICAL DUTIES:

LEGAL CONCEPTS

Practicum 22

_____	4. (c)	Apply principles of aseptic technique and infection control

Practicum 23

_____	4. (ff)	Perform telephone and in-person screening

Practicum 24

_____	4. (d)	Take vital signs
_____	5. (b)	Document accurately

Practicum 25

_____	2. (a)	Be attentive, listen, and learn
_____	2. (f)	Interview effectively
_____	2. (i)	Recognize and respond to verbal and nonverbal communication
_____	2. (j)	Use correct grammar, spelling and formatting techniques in written works.
_____	2. (k)	Principles of verbal and nonverbal communication
_____	2. (l)	Recognition and response to verbal and nonverbal communication
_____	4. (a)	Interview and take a patient history

_____   ***Total Points – Pass or Fail***

PROFESSIONALISM

CLINICAL DUTIES

COMMUNICATION

LEGAL CONCEPTS

Practicum 26

_____	1. (c)	Be a "team player"
_____	1. (e)	Exhibit initiative
_____	4. (g)	Prepare and maintain examination and treatment area

Practicum 27

_____	2. (b)	Be impartial and show empathy when dealing with patients
_____	2. (g)	Use appropriate medical terminology
_____	4. (h)	Assist physician with examinations and treatments
_____	4. (k)	Perform selected tests that assist with diagnosis and treatment
_____	4. (x)	Instruct patient in the collection of fecal specimen

Practicum 28

_____	4. (b)	Prepare patients for procedures
_____	4. (o)	Wrap items for autoclaving
_____	4. (p)	Perform sterilization techniques

Practicum 29

_____	4. (m)	Prepare and administer medications as directed by physicians - Oral

Practicum 30

_____	4. (m)	Prepare and administer medications as directed by physicians - Parenteral

Practicum 31

_____	4. (n)	Maintain medication records

Practicum 32

_____	4. (l)	Screen and follow up patient test results
_____	5. (h)	Perform risk management procedures

Practicum 33

_____	4. (q)	Dispose of biohazardous materials
_____	4. (r)	Practice standard precaution
_____	4. (s)	Perform venipuncture
_____	5. (b)	Document accurately

Practicum 34

_____	4. (j)	Collect and process specimens
_____	4. (t)	Perform capillary puncture
_____	4. (aa)	Perform chemistry testing
_____	4. (i)	Use quality control

Practicum 35

_____	4. (u)	Obtain throat specimen for microbiological testing
_____	4. (v)	Perform wound collection procedure for microbiological testing
_____	4. (cc)	Perform microbiology testing

Practicum 36

_____	4. (w)	Instruct patient in the collection of a clean-catch mid-stream urine specimen

Practicum 37

_____	4. (z)	Perform hematology

Practicum 38

_____	4. (bb)	Perform immunology testing

Practicum 39

_____	4. (i)	Use quality control
_____	4. (y)	Perform urinalysis

Practicum 40

_____	4. (dd)	Perform electrocardiograms
_____	5. (a)	Determine needs for documentation and reporting

Practicum 41

_____	4. (ee)	Perform respiratory testing

Practicum 42

_____	4. (e)	Recognize emergencies
_____	4. (f)	Perform first aid and CPR

_____   **Total Points – Pass or Fail**

The student named above:
_____ HAS achieved proficiency in the performance objectives.
_____ HAS NOT achieved proficiency in the performance objectives.

PART 2
Curriculum/Entry-Level Competencies

AAMA/CAAHEP Medical Assistant Curriculum/Entry-Level Competencies

1. Content

To provide for student attainment of the Entry-Level Competencies for the Medical Assistant, the curriculum must include as a minimum the following:

A. **ANATOMY AND PHYSIOLOGY**
   (1) Anatomy and physiology of all the body systems
   (2) Common pathology/diseases
   (3) Diagnostic/treatment modalities

B. **MEDICAL TERMINOLOGY**
   (1) Basic structure of medical words
   (2) Word building and definitions
   (3) Applications of medical terminology

C. **MEDICAL LAW AND ETHICS**
   (1) Legal guidelines/requirements for health care
   (2) Medical ethics and related issues

D. **PSYCHOLOGY**
   (1) Basic principles
   (2) Developmental stages of the life cycle
   (3) Hereditary, cultural, and environmental influences on behavior

E. **COMMUNICATION**
   (1) Principles of verbal and nonverbal communication
   (2) Recognition and response to verbal and nonverbal communication
   (3) Adaptations for individualized needs
   (4) Applications of electronic technology
   (5) Fundamental writing skills

F. **MEDICAL ASSISTING ADMINISTRATIVE PROCEDURES**
   (1) Basic medical assisting clerical functions
   (2) Bookkeeping principles
   (3) Insurance, procedural, and diagnostic coding
   (4) Operational functions

G. **MEDICAL ASSISTING CLINICAL PROCEDURES**
   (1) Asepsis and infection control
   (2) Specimen collection and processing
   (3) Diagnostic testing
   (4) Patient care
   (5) Pharmacology
   (6) Medical emergencies
   (7) Principles of IV therapy

H. **PROFESSIONAL COMPONENTS**
   (1) Personal attributes
   (2) Job readiness
   (3) Workplace dynamics
   (4) Allied health professions and credentialing
   (5) Provider level CPR certification and first aid training

2. Externship

A supervised, unpaid externship of at least 160 contact hours in an ambulatory health-care setting performing administrative and clinical procedures must be completed before graduation

3. Competencies

The Entry-Level Competencies for the medical assistant include, but are not limited to:

A. ADMINISTRATIVE COMPETENCIES

(1) Perform Clerical Functions
   a. Schedule and manage appointments
   b. Schedule inpatient and outpatient admissions and procedures
   c. Organize a patient's medical record
   d. File medical records

(2) Perform Bookkeeping Procedures
   a. Prepare a bank deposit
   b. Post entries on a day sheet
   c. Perform accounts receivable procedures
   d. Perform billing and collection procedures
   e. Post adjustments
   f. Process credit balance
   g. Process refunds
   h. Post NSF checks
   i. Post collection agency payments

(3) Process Insurance Claims
   a. Apply managed care policies and procedures
   b. Apply third-party guidelines
   c. Perform procedural coding
   d. Perform diagnostic coding
   e. Complete insurance claim forms

B. CLINICAL COMPETENCIES

(1) Fundamental Principles
   a. Perform hand washing
   b. Wrap items for autoclaving
   c. Perform sterilization techniques
   d. Dispose of biohazardous materials
   e. Practice Standard Precautions

(2) Specimen Collection
   a. Perform venipuncture
   b. Perform capillary puncture
   c. Obtain specimens for microbiological testing
   d. Instruct patients in the collection of a clean-catch mid-stream urine
   e. Instruct patients in the collection of fecal specimens

(3) Diagnostic Testing
   a. Perform electrocardiography
   b. Perform respiratory testing
   c. CLIA Waived Tests
      (i) Perform urinalysis
      (ii) Perform hematology testing
      (iii) Perform chemistry testing
      (iv) Perform immunology testing
      (v) Perform microbiology testing

(4) Patient Care
   a. Perform telephone and in-person screening
   b. Obtain vital signs
   c. Obtain and record patient history
   d. Prepare and maintain examination and treatment areas
   e. Prepare patient for and assist with routine and specialty examinations
   f. Prepare patient for and assist with procedures, treatments, and minor office surgeries
   g. Apply pharmacology principles to prepare and administer oral and parenteral (excluding IV) medications

    h. Maintain medication and immunization records
    i. Screen and follow-up test results

C. GENERAL COMPETENCIES

(1) Communicate
    a. Respond to and initiate written communications
    b. Recognize and respond to verbal communications
    c. Recognize and respond to nonverbal communications
    d. Demonstrate telephone techniques

(2) Legal Concepts
    a. Identify and respond to issues of confidentiality
    b. Perform within legal and ethical boundaries
    c. Establish and maintain the medical record
    d. Document appropriately
    e. Demonstrate knowledge of federal and state health care legislation and regulations

(3) Patient Instruction
    a. Explain general office policies
    b. Instruct individuals according to their needs
    c. Provide instruction for health maintenance and disease prevention
    d. Identify community resources

(4) Operational Functions
    a. Perform an inventory of supplies and equipment
    b. Perform routine maintenance of administrative and clinical equipment
    c. Utilize computer software to maintain office systems
    d. Use methods of quality control

AMT/ABHES Course Content and Competencies for Medical Assistants

1. Orientation
  A. INTRODUCTION AND REVIEW OF PROGRAM
    (1) Employment outlook
    (2) General responsibilities

2. Anatomy and Physiology
  A. ANATOMY AND PHYSIOLOGY
  B. DIET AND NUTRITION
  C. STUDY OF DISEASES AND ETIOLOGY
  D. ALL BODY SYSTEMS
  E. DIAGNOSTIC/TREATMENT MODALITIES

3. Medical Terminology
  A. BASIC STRUCTURE OF MEDICAL WORDS (ROOTS, PREFIXES, SUFFIXES, SPELLING, AND DEFINITIONS)
  B. COMBINING WORD ELEMENTS TO FORM MEDICAL WORDS
  C. MEDICAL SPECIALTIES AND SHORT FORMS
  D. MEDICAL ABBREVIATIONS

4. Medical Law and Ethics
  A. ETHICAL DECISIONS, MEDICAL JURISPRUDENCE AND CONFIDENTIALITY
  B. LEGAL TERMINOLOGY PERTAINING TO OFFICE PRACTICE
  C. MEDICAL/ETHICAL ISSUES IN TODAY'S SOCIETY
  D. RISK MANAGEMENT

5. Psychology of Human Relations
  A. DEALING WITH DIFFICULT PATIENTS WITH NORMAL/ABNORMAL BEHAVIOR
  B. CARING FOR PATIENTS WITH SPECIAL AND SPECIFIC NEEDS
  C. CARING FOR CANCER AND TERMINALLY ILL PATIENTS
  D. EMOTIONAL CRISES/PATIENTS AND/OR FAMILY
  E. VARIOUS TREATMENT PROTOCOLS
  F. BASIC PRINCIPLES
  G. DEVELOPMENTAL STAGES OF THE LIFE CYCLE
  H. HEREDITARY, CULTURAL, AND ENVIRONMENTAL INFLUENCES ON BEHAVIOR STANDARDS

6. Pharmacology
  A. OCCUPATIONAL MATH AND METRIC CONVERSIONS (DRUG CALCULATIONS)
  B. USE OF PDR AND MEDICATION BOOKS
  C. COMMON ABBREVIATIONS USED IN PRESCRIPTION WRITING

D. LEGAL ASPECTS OF WRITING PRESCRIPTIONS
E. FDC AND STATE LAWS
F. MEDICATIONS PRESCRIBED FOR THE TREATMENT OF ILLNESS AND DISEASE BASED ON A SYSTEMS METHOD

7. Medical Office Business Procedures/Management

A. MANUAL AND COMPUTERIZED RECORDS MANAGEMENT
   (1) Patient case histories (confidentiality)
   (2) Filing
   (3) Appointments and scheduling
   (4) Inventory/control
   (5) Financial management
   (6) Basic bookkeeping
   (7) Billing and collections
   (8) Purchasing
   (9) Banking and payroll
B. INSURANCE (INCLUDING HMOS, PPOS, CO-PAYS, CPT CODING, ETC.)
C. EQUIPMENT AND SUPPLIES (INCLUDING ORDERING/MAINTAINING/STORAGE/INVENTORY)
D. RECEPTION, PUBLIC AND INTERPERSONAL RELATIONS
   (1) Telephone techniques
   (2) Professional conduct and appearance
   (3) Professional office environment and safety
       a. Office safety and security

8. Basic Keyboarding

A. OFFICE MACHINES, TRANSCRIPTIONS, COMPUTERIZED SYSTEMS/MEDICAL DATA PROCESSING
B. TRANSCRIBING MEDICAL CORRESPONDENCE AND MEDICAL REPORTS
C. MEDICAL TERMINOLOGY REVIEW

9. Medical Office Clinical Procedures

A. BASIC CLINICAL SKILLS (E.G., VITAL SIGNS)
B. BASIC SKILLS AND PROCEDURES USED IN MEDICAL EMERGENCIES
C. PATIENT EXAMINATION
   (1) Patient histories
   (2) Patient preparation
   (3) Physical examination
   (4) Instruments
   (5) Assisting the physician
   (6) Housekeeping
D. MEDICAL EQUIPMENT
   (1) Electrocardiogram, centrifuge, etc.
   (2) Physical therapy
   (3) Radiography
       a. Safety
       b. Patient preparation
       c. Radiography of chest and extremities
E. MEDICAL ASEPSIS/STERILIZATION AND MINOR OFFICE SURGERY
F. SPECIALTIES
G. FIRST AID, CPR

H. INJECTIONS (DOSAGE CALCULATION)
    (1) IM
    (2) Subq
    (3) ID
I. UNIVERSAL PRECAUTIONS IN THE MEDICAL OFFICE

10. Medical Laboratory Procedures

A. ORIENTATION
    (1) Laboratory equipment and maintenance
    (2) Safety
    (3) Storage of chemicals and supplies
    (4) Fire safety
    (5) Care of microscope (introduction)
B. URINALYSIS
    (1) Specimen collection
    (2) Physical examination
    (3) Chemical analysis
    (4) Microscopic examination
C. HEMATOLOGY
    (1) Personal protective equipment
    (2) Specimen collection
        a. Venipuncture
        b. Finger puncture
    (3) Hemoglobin
    (4) Hematocrit
    (5) White blood cell (WBC)
    (6) Red blood cell (RBC)
    (7) Slide preps
    (8) Serology
        a. Blood typing
        b. Blood morphology
    (9) Quality control
D. BASIC BLOOD CHEMISTRIES
E. HIV/AIDS AND BLOODBORNE PATHOGENS
F. OSHA COMPLIANCE RULES AND REGULATIONS

11. Career Development

A. INSTRUCTION REGARDING INTERNSHIP RULES, REGULATION
B. JOB SEARCH, PROFESSIONAL DEVELOPMENT, AND SUCCESS
C. GOAL SETTING, TIME MANAGEMENT, EMPLOYMENT OPPORTUNITIES
D. RESUME WRITING, INTERVIEWING TECHNIQUES, AND FOLLOW-UP
E. DRESS FOR SUCCESS
F. PROFESSIONALISM

12. Guidelines for Acceptable Externship (160 Hours)

A. THE EXTERNSHIP SHOULD PROVIDE STUDENTS PRACTICAL
    EXPERIENCE IN AMBULATORY HEALTH CARE FACILITIES, INCLUDING
    HOSPITALS, PHYSICIAN'S OFFICES, OR OTHER HEALTH CARE
    FACILITIES.
B. BEFORE ASSIGNING A STUDENT TO AN EXTERNSHIP LOCATION, THERE
    MUST BE A PRIOR EVALUATION BY THE SCHOOL THAT A VIABLE

EXTERNSHIP SITE EXISTS FOR AN EFFECTIVE EXTERNSHIP. IN ADDITION, THE PHYSICIAN SHALL BE PROVIDED WITH A WRITTEN CONTRACT SETTING FORTH THE CONDITIONS FOR THE EXTERNSHIP.

C. VISITATION BY A QUALIFIED MEMBER OF THE SCHOOL STAFF SHOULD BE MADE DURING THE EXTERNSHIP OF A TRAINEE IF THE LOCALE IS WITHIN A REASONABLE DISTANCE FROM THE SCHOOL. IN ANY EVENT, TELEPHONE FOLLOW-UP SHOULD BE MADE TO DETERMINE THAT THE EXPERIENCE IS A VALID AND SATISFACTORY ONE FOR THE TRAINEE.

D. THE EXTERNSHIP SHOULD INCLUDE APPROPRIATELY DIVERSIFIED LEARNING EXPERIENCES.

E. A DOCUMENTED REPORT ON STUDENT PERFORMANCE MUST BE SUBMITTED BY THE PHYSICIAN AND/OR THE SUPERVISORY PERSON INVOLVED. THE REPORT MUST BE KEPT AT THE SCHOOL IN THE STUDENT'S FILE.

Entry-Level Competencies

Competencies required for successful completion of the program shall be clearly delineated.

1. Professionalism
    A. PROJECT A POSITIVE ATTITUDE
    B. MAINTAIN CONFIDENTIALITY AT ALL TIMES
    C. BE A "TEAM PLAYER"
    D. BE COGNIZANT OF ETHICAL BOUNDARIES
    E. EXHIBIT INITIATIVE
    F. ADAPT TO CHANGE
    G. EVIDENCE A RESPONSIBLE ATTITUDE
    H. BE COURTEOUS AND DIPLOMATIC
    I. CONDUCT WORK WITHIN SCOPE OF EDUCATION, TRAINING, AND ABILITY

2. Communication
    A. BE ATTENTIVE, LISTEN, AND LEARN
    B. BE IMPARTIAL AND SHOW EMPATHY WHEN DEALING WITH PATIENTS
    C. ADAPT WHAT IS SAID TO THE RECIPIENT'S LEVEL OF COMPREHENSION
    D. SERVE AS LIAISON BETWEEN PHYSICIAN AND OTHERS
    E. USE PROPER TELEPHONE TECHNIQUES
    F. INTERVIEW EFFECTIVELY
    G. USE APPROPRIATE MEDICAL TERMINOLOGY
    H. RECEIVE, ORGANIZE, PRIORITIZE, AND TRANSMIT INFORMATION EXPEDIENTLY
    I. RECOGNIZE AND RESPOND TO VERBAL AND NONVERBAL COMMUNICATION
    J. USE CORRECT GRAMMAR, SPELLING, AND FORMATTING TECHNIQUES IN WRITTEN WORKS
    K. PRINCIPLES OF VERBAL AND NONVERBAL COMMUNICATION
    L. RECOGNITION AND RESPONSE TO VERBAL AND NONVERBAL COMMUNICATION
    M. ADAPTATION FOR INDIVIDUALIZED NEEDS
    N. APPLICATION OF ELECTRONIC TECHNOLOGY
    O. FUNDAMENTAL WRITING SKILLS
    P. PROFESSIONAL COMPONENTS
    Q. ALLIED HEALTH PROFESSIONS AND CREDENTIALING

3. Administrative Duties
    A. PERFORM BASIC SECRETARIAL SKILLS
    B. PREPARE AND MAINTAIN MEDICAL RECORDS
    C. SCHEDULE AND MONITOR APPOINTMENTS
    D. APPLY COMPUTER CONCEPTS FOR OFFICE PROCEDURES
    E. PERFORM MEDICAL TRANSCRIPTION
    F. LOCATE RESOURCES AND INFORMATION FOR PATIENTS AND EMPLOYERS

G. MANAGE PHYSICIAN'S PROFESSIONAL SCHEDULE AND TRAVEL
H. SCHEDULE INPATIENT AND OUTPATIENT ADMISSIONS
I. PREPARE A BANK STATEMENT
J. POST ENTRIES ON A DAY SHEET
K. RECONCILE A BANK STATEMENT
L. POST ENTRIES ON A DAY SHEET
M. PERFORM BILLING AND COLLECTION PROCEDURES
N. PREPARE A CHECK
O. ESTABLISH AND MAINTAIN A PETTY CASH FUND
P. POST ADJUSTMENTS
Q. PROCESS CREDIT BALANCE
R. PROCESS REFUNDS
S. POST NSF FUNDS
T. POST COLLECTION AGENCY PAYMENTS
U. APPLY MANAGED CARE POLICIES AND PROCEDURES
V. OBTAIN MANAGED CARE REFERRALS AND PRECERTIFICATION
W. PERFORM DIAGNOSTIC CODING
X. COMPLETE INSURANCE CLAIM FORMS
Y. USE PHYSICIAN FEE SCHEDULE

4. Clinical Duties

A. INTERVIEW AND TAKE PATIENT HISTORY
B. PREPARE PATIENTS FOR PROCEDURES
C. APPLY PRINCIPLES OF ASEPTIC TECHNIQUES AND INFECTION CONTROL
D. TAKE VITAL SIGNS
E. RECOGNIZE EMERGENCIES
F. PERFORM FIRST AID AND CPR
G. PREPARE AND MAINTAIN EXAMINATION AND TREATMENT AREA
H. ASSIST PHYSICIAN WITH EXAMINATIONS AND TREATMENTS
I. USE QUALITY CONTROL
J. COLLECT AND PROCESS SPECIMENS
K. PERFORM SELECTED TESTS THAT ASSIST WITH DIAGNOSIS AND TREATMENT
L. SCREEN AND FOLLOW UP PATIENT TEST RESULTS
M. PREPARE AND ADMINISTER MEDICATIONS AS DIRECTED BY PHYSICIAN
N. MAINTAIN MEDICATION RECORDS
O. WRAP ITEMS FOR AUTOCLAVING
P. PERFORM STERILIZATION TECHNIQUES
Q. DISPOSE OF BIOHAZARDOUS MATERIALS
R. PRACTICE STANDARD PRECAUTIONS
S. PERFORM VENIPUNCTURE
T. PERFORM CAPILLARY PUNCTURE
U. OBTAIN THROAT SPECIMEN FOR MICROBIOLOGICAL TESTING
V. PERFORM WOUND COLLECTION PROCEDURE FOR MICROBIOLOGICAL TESTING

W. INSTRUCT PATIENTS IN THE COLLECTION OF A CLEAN-CATCH MID-STREAM URINE SPECIMEN
X. INSTRUCT PATIENT IN THE COLLECTION OF FECAL SPECIMEN
Y. PERFORM URINALYSIS
Z. PERFORM HEMATOLOGY
AA. PERFORM CHEMISTRY TESTING
BB. PERFORM IMMUNOLOGY TESTING
CC. PERFORM MICROBIOLOGY TESTING
DD. PERFORM ELECTROCARDIOGRAMS
EE. PERFORM RESPIRATORY TESTING
FF. PERFORM TELEPHONE AND IN-PERSON SCREENING

5. Legal Concepts

A. DETERMINE NEEDS FOR DOCUMENTATION AND REPORTING
B. DOCUMENT ACCURATELY
C. USE APPROPRIATE GUIDELINES WHEN RELEASING RECORDS OR INFORMATION
D. FOLLOW ESTABLISHED POLICY IN INITIATING OR TERMINATING MEDICAL TREATMENT
E. DISPOSE OF CONTROLLED SUBSTANCES IN COMPLIANCE WITH GOVERNMENT REGULATIONS
F. MAINTAIN LICENSES AND ACCREDITATION
G. MONITOR LEGISLATION RELATED TO CURRENT HEALTH-CARE ISSUES AND PRACTICES
H. PERFORM RISK MANAGEMENT PROCEDURES

6. Office Management

A. MAINTAIN PHYSICAL PLANT
B. OPERATE AND MAINTAIN FACILITIES AND EQUIPMENT SAFELY
C. INVENTORY EQUIPMENT AND SUPPLIES
D. EVALUATE AND RECOMMEND EQUIPMENT AND SUPPLIES FOR PRACTICE
E. MAINTAIN LIABILITY COVERAGE
F. EXERCISE EFFICIENT TIME MANAGEMENT

7. Instruction

A. ORIENT PATIENTS TO OFFICE POLICIES AND PROCEDURES
B. INSTRUCT PATIENTS WITH SPECIAL NEEDS
C. TEACH PATIENTS METHODS OF HEALTH PROMOTION AND DISEASE PREVENTION
D. ORIENT AND TRAIN PERSONNEL

8. Financial Management

A. USE MANUAL AND COMPUTERIZED BOOKKEEPING SYSTEMS
B. IMPLEMENT CURRENT PROCEDURAL TERMINOLOGY AND ICD-9 CODING

C. ANALYZE AND USE CURRENT THIRD-PARTY GUIDELINES FOR REIMBURSEMENT
D. MANAGE ACCOUNTS PAYABLE AND RECEIVABLE
E. MAINTAIN RECORDS FOR ACCOUNTING AND BANKING PURPOSES
F. PROCESS EMPLOYEE PAYROLL

PART 3
Database

Physician Information

Dr. Franklin Pierce Wright, Family Practice
2310 Wright Way
Melbourne, FL 32904
Telephone (904) 565-3200

State License Number	#G46789
UPIN #	#5890187340
Tax ID#	#59-8710766
DEA#	#9151489890

Message Services

Coastal Answering Service	#73-AM messages	#72-PM service
Dr. Wright's Beeper	#435-7177	
Dr. Wright's Cell Phone	#787-1199	

Office Hours

Monday–Thursday 8:30 AM–5: 30 PM
Closed for Lunch 1:00–2:00 PM
Friday 9:00 AM –1:00 PM

CLOSED FOR THE FOLLOWING HOLIDAYS (MATRIX)

Good Friday
Memorial Day
Labor Day
Christmas Eve and Day
Thanksgiving Thursday and Friday

Philosophy: Principles and Professional Conduct

PRINCIPLES

- Make a Difference
- Associate and Team Effort Development
- Accountability for the Community
- Pricing that Is Competitive
- Clientele Satisfaction
- Integrated Services
- Physician Leadership
- Quality Health Care

PROFESSIONAL CONDUCT

It is the philosophy and professional conduct of this office to provide the highest quality of care while maintaining the dignity and individuality of all persons who enter this medical office. This practice is founded on a common set of values that govern our relationship with our patients, fellow physicians, third-party payers and providers, vendors, consultants, and one another. We pride ourselves on integrity, honesty, and fairness. The physician and staff are dedicated to meeting the health needs of our patients through quality and competency while insuring the patient's equal rights. The goal of this office is to apply the highest legal and ethical principles in carrying out all office procedures and policies. This practice will also strive to "Make a Difference" in all aspects of your health care and your individuality.

HIPAA

Health Insurance Portability and Accountability Act of 1996 (HIPAA) and Patient Confidentiality are maintained in this office completely and at all times. All new patients are required to complete the following forms:

- Patient Profile/Past Medical History
- New Patient Information/Insurance
- Acknowledgment of Receipt of Notice of Privacy Practices
- ABN (Advanced Beneficiary Notice's)
- Consent to the Use and Disclosure of Health Information for Treatment, Payment, or Health Care Operations

We obtain medical information in the course of our duties that is sensitive. By its very nature, it concerns inherently personal and private aspects of our patients' lives. Given the sensitive nature of the information, it is the policy of this practice to treat all patient information with the utmost discretion and confidentiality and to prohibit improper release in accordance with requirement of state and Federal laws.

The Health Insurance Portability and Accountability Act of 1996 (August 21), Public Law 104-191, which amends the Internal Revenue Service Code of 1986, is also known as the Kennedy-Kassebaum Act. Title II of this act includes a section, Administrative Simplification, which was implemented to improve efficiency in health-care delivery by standardizing electronic data interchange and to protect the confidentiality and security of health data through setting and enforcing standards.

HIPAA calls for the standardization of electronic patient health, administrative, and financial data; unique health identifiers for individuals, employers, health plans, and health-care providers; and security standards protecting the confidentiality and integrity of "individually identifiable health information," past, present, or future.

All health-care organizations, and other organizations are affected by this law, including physicians, health plans, employers, public health authorities, life insurers, clearing houses, billing agencies, information system vendors, service organizations, and universities.

Remember that HIPAA calls for severe civil and criminal penalties for noncompliance, including fines up to $25,000 for multiple violation of the same standard in a calendar year and fines up to $250,000 and/or imprisonment up to 10 years for knowing misuse of individually identifiable health information.

Chart Policy/Contents

- All New Patient forms (Demographics, Insurance, and HIPAA) are to be kept on the left side of chart
- Chart is tabbed with sections – All notes or other medical correspondence is to be kept on the right side of the chart in Reverse Chronological order.
- Problem List/Progress Notes
- Medication List
- Nonroutine Disclosure Log

Employees

- To maintain quality of care and adhere to standards, Dr. Wright only employs licensed or certified/registered health care employees. Human resources will verify and keep current copies of all/each employee's credentials. As an employee of this office, you are expected to keep current any and all continuing education units required to maintain your credentialed status. An educational allowance of $150.00 per year will be available to help defray the continuing education costs.
- Employees will receive Performance Evaluations by Dr. Wright biyearly, at which time your strengths and weaknesses will be discussed. You will be given a 90-day notice for areas requiring improvement and will be reevaluated.
- All employees are required to read the Policy and Procedural Manuals and sign the form that they understand the rules and regulations set forth by this practice and will practice these rules and policies.
- All In-services for HIPAA, OSHA, Tuberculosis, AIDS, and Bloodborne Pathogens will be provided by this facility, and a copy of your current certificate will be kept in your employee file.
- All employee files are kept confidential.

- It is the responsibility of the employee to become familiar with all forms associated with this practice.
- Employee benefits, vacation and sick leave, hourly wages, and withholding will be explained to the employee on the first day of hiring.
- Our employees are expected to work as a team. Although there will be specific employee assignments and job duties, we are all here to assist the patient and the physician in any way possible.

Physician Preferences

- Hospital Rounds: 7:00-8:00 AM
- Appointments: Schedule Complete Physicals (new patient [NP]/established patient [EP]) and Well-baby visits in morning. Allow 1 hour for Complete Physicals

ON-CALL PHYSICIANS

Dr. Biggiot   Beeper #453-9002   Office: 453-2265
Dr. Schiffer   Beeper #457-9080   Office: 457-1288

Accepts Assignment (AA)/Provider	Provider #
Medicare	#Z678234190
Medicaid	#12367800034
Aetna	#9476202556
Blue Cross and Blue Shield (BC/BS)	#7341008547
Prudential	#2108874652
Tricare	#997865446

Financial Procedures

ACCOUNTS RECEIVABLE

The office uses manual and medical computer software for accounts payable and receivable. Charges and payments will be entered in the computer and on the pegboard, including the physician charge slip, patient ledger card, and the day sheet.

PAYMENTS

Before a patient's visit, the fees and insurance are to be discussed with the patient. Payment is due after services are rendered (co-pay, deductible, or percentage due).

The office will file insurance on all patients at no charge regardless whether we are a provider or not.

BANKING

Deposits are made every Monday, Wednesday, and Friday. Bank statements are to be reconciled monthly. Checking Account #: 11500040085. All checks for deposit must be stamped with "For Deposit Only."

BILLING

Patients with account balances will be billed on the 15th (A–M) and 30th (N–Z) of each month. Maintain computer and manual records.

COLLECTIONS

Policy for collections of delinquent accounts is as follows:

- Accounts 30 days past due – Cycle Billing
- Accounts 60 days past due – Cycle Billing/Phone call
- Accounts 90 days past due – Cycle Billing/Collection Letter
- Accounts 120 days or more past due – Send to Collections

Collect Collection Agency
54 Nuber Drive
Tampa, FL 98452

INSURANCE CARRIERS

Verify coverage for all new and established patients. Patients with Medicaid cards will be verified each visit. Obtain authorization and/or precertification for all procedures, including Outpatient and Inpatient services. File all claims the same day of the service.

REFERRALS

Referrals are completed by this office as a courtesy to the patient. Obtain the referral number from the insured's insurance company and complete the referral form. As a courtesy, we will also assist in setting up the referral appointment.

ACCOUNTS PAYABLE

All vendors will be paid within the discount period. All other invoices will be paid by the 5th and 20th of the month. Employees are paid weekly on Fridays after 3:00 PM. Payroll journal, check register, and distribution journal will be proofed and balanced at the end of each business day. The accounts receivable and payable journals will be totaled and balanced at the end of each month and prepared for the accountant quarterly.

Daily Procedure Manual

LABORATORY STATIONS

- All items stocked neatly. First In Last Out if applicable
- All countertops wiped with disinfectant
- All phlebotomy chairs and stations disinfected
- All trash, sharps, or biohazard materials in appropriate containers
- All items have been removed from the cold sterile and replaced

EXAMINATION/TREATMENT AREAS

- All examination tables disinfected and clean table paper applied
- Attached or loose stools swept and cleaned
- Weight scales swept and cleaned
- All mayo jars and canisters stocked
- All equipment cleaned and maintained in appropriate compartments
- All thermometers cleaned and stored properly
- All patient education forms replenished

SINK/SURGICAL ASEPTIC – NONSURGICAL ASEPTIC AREA

- All items removed from cold sterile
- All sinks cleaned and stocked with new paper towels
- All soap and disinfectant containers refilled for use
- All instruments put back where they belong
- All countertops disinfected and wiped dry

I, _____, as an employee of Dr. Wright's have been informed of the above office policy and daily procedures. I have read and understand all of the above and will abide by these rules to ensure a sound, secure, and safe workplace and environment.

_____   _____
Employee (Student) Signature   Date

List of Dr. Wright's Patients

DEMOGRAPHIC INFORMATION

INSURANCE/DEPENDENT INFORMATION

Name: Sandra Backer   **DOB:** 09-30-42
Address: 18 Mulberry St.   **SS#:** 265-67-9010
Palmetto, FL 90256   **Tel (H):** 512-453-6767
Insurance: Medicare   **Emp:** Retired
ID#: 265679010C   **Tel(W):** NA
Group#: NA   **Spouse:** NA
Pre-Cert#: MC8944-Covered

Name: Ethel Burke   **DOB:** 04-25-25
Address: 546 Dustin Ave.   **SS#:** 629-98-6301
Surfside, FL 90867   **Tel (H):** 568-321-7356
Insurance: Medicare   **Emp:** Retired
ID#: 629986301C   **Tel(W):** NA
Group#: 61842   **Spouse:** Samuel 11-21-24
   SS#: 510-52-7350

Name: Antonio Cann   **DOB:** 10-20-27
Address: 2300 Ocean Way   **SS#:** 438-00-7810
Surfside, FL 90866   **Tel (H):** 561-778-7329
Insurance: Medicare   **Emp:** Retired
ID#: 438007810C   **Tel(W):** NA
Group#: 45001   **Spouse:** Franchesca 11-14-30
   SS#: 719-41-7830

Name:	Ann Curt	**DOB:**	03-21-61
Address:	31 Shore Dr.	**SS#:**	161-76-0606
	Surfside, FL 90866	**Tel (H):**	568-321-7891
Insurance:	Prudential	**Emp:**	Carter Vision Center
	ID#: 3861409862	**Tel(W):**	907-568-3434
	Group#: 61984	**Spouse:**	Ronald 06-11-62
		SS#:	610-71-5630

Name:	Dan Had	**DOB:**	05-21-73
Address:	571 East St.	**SS#:**	519-52-7164
	Palm Coast, FL 90168	**Tel (H):**	907 561-6523
Insurance:	Aetna	**Emp:**	Harr Electronics
	ID#: NA	**Tel(W):**	906-568-6190
	Group#: 61893	**Spouse:**	Karan 09-17-73
		SS#:	459-61-5398
		Dependents:	Justin DOB: 11-13-96
			Joanne DOB: 08-24-97
			Jennifer DOB: 01-25-98
			Jake DOB: 05-04-00

Name:	Kris Hardee	**DOB:**	01-31-66
Address:	678 Garver St.	**SS#:**	768-01-8732
	Palm Coast, FL 90167	**Tel (H):**	907-676-3214
Insurance:	Blue Cross/Blue Shield	**Emp:**	Excel College
	ID#: NA	**Tel(W):**	512-546-1313
	Group#: 67110	**Spouse:**	Pat 01-30-64
		SS#:	368-90-6564

Name:	Quint Jonas	**DOB:**	03-30-35
Address:	56 Archer St.	**SS#:**	629-91-8329
	Palmetto, FL 90257	**Tel (H):**	561-568-0343
Insurance:	Medicare	**Emp:**	Retired
	ID#: 629918329B	**Tel(W):**	NA
	Group#: 61947	**Spouse:**	Helen 11-14-36
		SS#:	510-73-7153

Name:	Neil Kaine	**DOB:**	12-23-47
Address:	710 Dolphin St.	**SS#:**	672-94-6382
	Palmetto, FL 90257	**Tel (H):**	517-562-8365
Insurance:	Prudential	**Emp:**	Kaine Dry Cleaning
	ID#: 9163064539	**Tel(W):**	517-568-9000
	Group#: 73541	**Spouse:**	Yoko 01-15-47
		SS#:	845-29-8210

Name:	Mary Manygrats	**DOB:**	02-20-45
Address:	980 Fern St.	**SS#:**	983-01-6385
	Palmetto, FL 90257	**Tel (H):**	512-777-2648
Insurance:	Prudential	**Emp:**	Carol's Hair Salon
	ID#: 2096482105	**Tel(W):**	512-779-2323
	Group#: 86206	**Spouse:**	Jim 06-11-44
		SS#:	267-81-5834

Name: Sheley Minton   **DOB:** 11-06-97
Address: 3110 Coral Reef Way   **SS#:** 362-71-7350
Palm Coast, FL 90169   **Guardian:** Mariah Minton
Insurance: Prudential   **Tel (H):** 907-562-7198
ID#: 3901835104   **Emp:** Flowers by Rose
Group#: 19640   **Tel(W):** 907-568-9292
SS#: 108-56-3876

Name: Dan Olstine   **DOB:** 11-22-02
Address: 3231 Sunshine Skyway   **SS#:** 345-678-9111
Palm Coast, FL 90167   **Guardian:** Janice Ovelbe
Insurance: Prudential   **Tel (H):** 904-777-3161
ID#: 8075467100   **Tel(W):** 904-778-8112
Group#: 56003   **SS#:** 611 05 9000

Name: Marcus Plan   **DOB:** 10-08-29
Address: 450 Windemere Pl.   **SS#:** 297-73-2784
Palm Coast, FL 90169   **Tel (H):** 907-286-5672
Insurance: Medicare   **Emp:** Retired
ID#: 297732784A   **Tel(W):** NA
Group#: 72195   **Spouse:** Audra 09-22-31
SS#: 490-38-1298

Name: Patty Quint **DOB:** 03-28-71
Address: 60 Hibiscus Ct. **SS#:** 483-81-5830
Surfside, FL 90866 **Tel (H):** 561-568-3810
Insurance: Blue Cross/Blue Shield **Emp:** Bonns Realestate
ID#: 3901743829 **Tel(W):** 907-561-8181
Group#: 49015 **Spouse:** William 09-08-70
SS#: 109-45-8267

Name: Patrice Roc **DOB:** 12-23-59
Address: 1425 Wave Ave. **SS#:** 367-75-3150
Surfside, FL 90867 **Tel (H):** 561-983-5457
Insurance: Aetna **Emp:** Florida Electric
ID#: NA **Tel(W):** 561-222-0101
Group#: 78312 **Spouse:** Jeff DOB: 06-07-60
SS#: 245-90-9984
Dependents: Andrea DOB: 08-04-87
Abigail DOB: 09-24-89

Name: Darcee Rooso **DOB:** 01-28-67
Address: 2121 Sheridan Pl. **SS#:** 639-10-8237
Surfside, FL 90867 **Tel (H):** 561-985-5451
Insurance: Prudential **Emp:** Porter House
ID#: 1046825900 **Tel(W):** 907-779-3967
Group#: 20582 **Spouse:** Neil James 07-10-66
Precertification #: 4890288dy **SS#:** 984-81-46

Name: Lindy Schaffer **DOB:** 09-15-97
Address: 4300 Kerrigan St. **SS#:** 768-01-8732
Palmetto, FL 90256 **Guardian:** Mary Schaffer
Insurance: Aetna **Tel (H):** 512-779-4321
ID#: NA **Emp:** Paramount Inc.
Group#: 88280 **Tel(W):** 907- 778-3300
SS#: 487-91-3895

Name: Ken Slate **DOB:** 02-13-42
Address: 3456 Palms Ave. **SS#:** 161-78-0770
Palm Coast, FL 90167 **Tel (H):** 904-778-3211
Insurance: Aetna **Emp:** Pride and Country
ID#: 9013257824 **Tel(W):** 904-787-5435
Group#: 90908 **Spouse:** Mary Slate 08 15 45

Name: Dennis Stine **DOB:** 08-10-77
Address: 3434 Burch St. **SS#:** 420-78-6310
Palmetto, FL 90256 **Tel (H):** 561-567-5061
Insurance: Blue Cross/ Blue Shield **Emp:** Cosmos Hair
ID#: 1290765430 **Tel(W):** 561-568-0090
Group#: 495201 **Spouse:** NA

Name: Ernest Swain   **DOB:** 05-10-99
Address: 4150 Harbor Dr.   **SS#:** 845-72-7634
Palm Coast, FL 90169   **Guardian:** Dennis Swain
Insurance: Tricare   **Tel (H):** 907-568-9016
ID#: NA   **Emp:** Commerce Trucking
Group#: 73916   **Tel(W):** 321-453-2121
SS#: 832-71-7309

Name: Debby Verisso   **DOB:** 04-21-35
Address: 6767 Palmetto Dr.   **SS#:** 598-01-2267
Palm Coast, FL 90168   **Tel (H):** 907-778-6787
Insurance: Medicare   **Emp:** Retired
ID#: 598012267B   **Tel(W):** NA
Spouse: Dannee 02-14-36
SS#: 003-67-1259

Fee Service/Schedule

FEE – SERVICE

Level E/M #		Time	Fee

OFFICE VISIT/ NEW (NP)

Code	Description	Time	Fee
99201*	Focused	10 minutes	$45.00
99202	Expanded	20 minutes	$50.00
99203	Detailed	30 minutes	$65.00
99204	Comprehensive	45 minutes	$95.00
99205	Complex	60 minutes	$150.00

OFFICE VISIT/ ESTABLISHED (EP)

Code	Description	Time	Fee
99211	Minimal	5 minutes	$40.00
99212	Focused	10 minutes	$45.00
99213	Expanded	15 minutes	$50.00
99214	Detailed	25 minutes	$65.00
99215	Comprehensive	40 minutes	$95.00

OFFICE PROCEDURES

Code	Description	Fee
93000	ECG 12 Lead	$55.00
93015	ECG, Treadmill	$295.00
92551	Audiometry Screen	$15.00
10060	I&D	$45.00
11400	Excision-Lesion 0.5 cm or less	$25.00/cm
12001	Laceration Repair 2.5 cm or less	$25.00/cm
11730	Nail Removal	$45.00
94010	Spirometry	$50.00
69210	Cerumen Removal (Ear Lavage)	$40.00

LABORATORY

Code	Description	Fee
99000	Collection/Handling Laboratory Specimen	$10.00
36415	Venipuncture	$10.00
85027	CBC	$25.00
85014	Hematocrit	$10.00
85018	Hemoglobin	$10.00
85002	Bleeding Time	$25.00
82948	Glucose/Reagent Strip	$10.00
82951	GTT	$75.00
81000	Urinalysis	$20.00
81002	Urinalysis (Dip Only)	$12.00
81025	Urine Pregnancy Test/Visual Color	$10.00
87081	Culture/Strep Throat	$10.00
87060	Culture, Throat	$25.00
88150-90	PAP (Outside Lab)	$12.00

INJECTIONS AND IMMUNIZATIONS

90707	MMR	$25.00
90712	OPV	$25.00
90701	DTP	$25.00
90647	Hib	$20.00
90658	Influenza Injection	$20.00
90732	Pneumococcal Injection	$20.00
90788	Antibiotic (IM)	$25.00

OFFICE X-RAY

73000	Clavicle	$50.00
73030-22	Shoulder/3 Views	$75.00
73090	Forearm	$75.00
73110	Wrist	$75.00
73610	Ankle	$50.00
71020	Chest/2 Views	$50.00

*Examples of Procedural Codes; subject to change per year; Students may also look codes up in the current year Current Procedural Terminology (CPT) book if available.

Common Diagnosis Codes

Otitis Media, Acute	382.9*	Well-Child Health Examination	V20.2
Chronic	382.9	Well-Adult Health Examination	V70.9
Asthma, Bronchial	493.9	Conjunctivitis/Acute	372.00
w/COPD	493.2	Cystitis/Acute	595.0
Fungus Nail	110.1	Urinary Tract Infection	5.990
Allergic,w/SA	493.91	Streptococcal Infection	041.00
Allergic,w/o SA	493.90	Anemia	285.9
Hypertension, Malignant	401.0	Diabetes	250.0 (see ICD-9 for modifiers)
Benign	401.1	Fracture Ankle Closed	824.8
Unspecified	401.9	Fracture Clavicle Closed	810.0
w/CHF	402.91	Fracture Forearm Closed	813.80
Ischemic Heart Disease	414.9	Fracture Humerus Upper End	812.00
w/o MI	411.89	Fracture Wrist Closed	814.00
w/Coronary Occlusion	411.81		

*Examples of Common Diagnosis Codes; subject to change each year; Students can also look up codes in current year ICD-9 book.

Laboratories Used by Physician/Insurance Companies

BAYSIDE LABORATORY

388 Shores Dr.
Melbourne, FL 32940
800 432-9066

QUALITY CONTROL GUARANTEED LABORATORY

45 Millside Ave.
Melbourne, FL 32941
800 432-7731

PART 4
Administrative Competencies

Practicum 1. Adapting to Change

COMPETENCY

CAAHEP: NA
ABHES: 1. (f) Adapt to change

SPECIFIC TASK

Using the scenario below and role-playing with a classmate show your professionalism by explaining how you can adapt to change. Your fellow classmate will play as the office manager.

STANDARD PRECAUTIONS

NA

EQUIPMENT/SUPPLIES

Pen

STANDARD OF PERFORMANCE OF THE TASK

You may earn a maximum of 5 points for each competency regardless of the number of steps to be performed.

   EX: If you miss two steps and achieve all the rest then you have earned 3 points.
   More than five steps missed means that you have 0 points.
   Your instructor may choose not to assign points but check you off on a pass or fail status.
Regardless, you may need to repeat the competency for successful completion.
   It is up to your instructor to determine the maximum number of tries before the competency has been met successfully in the time allotted

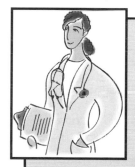

Make a Difference

Many times through your employment you will be asked by the supervisor, office manager, or physician to perform a task or duty that is not normally in your job description. We all want to work as a team and be flexible when needed even though the task asked of you might not be something that you like doing. This is one of the great aspects about the profession of Medical Assisting; you are a multi-tasked individual. Always show how you are willing to act as a team member, show professionalism, and adapt to change by accepting any new assignment that may come your way.

Student Name: _____   Date: _____

Time: Satisfactory   Unsatisfactory

Successful Completion: Yes   No

Grade/Points: _____   Pass   Fail

Need to Repeat: _____   Number of Attempts: 1   2   3

Instructor Comments: _____

_____

_____

CONDITIONS UNDER WHICH THE STUDENT IS EXPECTED TO PERFORM THE TASK

Follow Task/Performance Steps

Task/Performance Step	S	U
1. Student listens attentively as physician asks employee to perform a different role this week.		
2. Student graciously and positively offers to help in any capacity where help is needed.		
3. Student documented how he/she can positively and professionally adapt to change when needed.		

SMART THINKING

Your office is shorthanded this week. It is flu season and one of the front office employees is not able to make it to work.

Normally, you work in the back office and perform all the clinical duties by assisting the physician. This week the physician asks you if you will work in the front office and fill in for the employee who is out sick. He asks that you schedule appointments, pull charts, file, and assist others in the front office when asked to perform other tasks associated with the reception area.

Document below how you will graciously and professionally adapt to this change and what your response to the physician will be.

_____

_____

_____

_____

_____

_____

_____

Practicum 2. Confidentiality

COMPETENCY

CAAHEP: 3. c. (2) (a) Identify and respond to issues of confidentiality
ABHES: 1. (b) Maintain confidentiality at all times
             5. (c) Use appropriate guidelines when releasing records or information

SPECIFIC TASK

Below you will find two scenarios that have breached patient confidentiality and HIPAA in your office. Correct the scenarios by addressing what could have been done to ensure it won't happen in the future and confidentiality will be maintained. Role-play with a classmate for any forms that you feel are necessary to prevent this in the future.

STANDARD PRECAUTIONS

NA

EQUIPMENT/SUPPLIES

Included case scenario
Black pen
HIPAA forms (attached)
Medical Record Release (attached)

STANDARD OF PERFORMANCE OF THE TASK

You may earn a maximum of 5 points for each competency regardless of the number of steps to be performed.
    EX: If you miss two steps and achieve all the rest then you have earned 3 points.
    More than five steps missed means that you have 0 points.
    Your instructor may choose not to assign points but check you off on a pass or fail status.
Regardless, you may need to repeat the competency for successful completion.
    It is up to your instructor to determine the maximum number of tries before the competency has been met successfully in the time allotted.

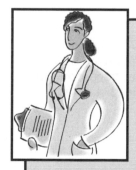

Make a Difference

Protecting patient confidentiality is a serious issue. Part of the Medical Assistant Creed states, "I protect the confidence entrusted to me." There is a national standard known as HIPAA (Health Insurance Portability and Accountability Act of 1996) that was enacted by the federal government and protects patients' personal health information from inappropriate disclosure and use. This set of rules ensures the privacy of the patients. Always have the patient's written consent for releasing information. Always ensure that the patient has completed the proper HIPAA forms.

Student Name: _____   Date: _____

Time: Satisfactory   Unsatisfactory

Successful Completion: Yes   No

Grade/Points: _____   Pass   Fail

Need to Repeat: _____   Number of Attempts: 1   2   3

Instructor Comments: _____

_____

_____

CONDITIONS UNDER WHICH THE STUDENT IS EXPECTED TO PERFORM THE TASK

Follow Task/Performance Steps

Task/Performance Step	S	U
1. Student correctly identified the problem. *Health-care employees should never discuss patient information unless it pertains to the treatment and care of the patient.*		
2. Student addressed guidelines and standards on how to avoid this type of scenario in the future.		
3. Student correctly identified the nature of the problem. *Had the patient completed the appropriate HIPAA and Medical Record Release forms this would have never happened.*		
4. Student discussed and completed the appropriate forms with patient.		

Key: Satisfactory = S; Unsatisfactory = U

SMART THINKING

SCENARIO #1

A patient is taken into an examination room and informs the medical assistant that she overheard a conversation between two of the receptionists talking about a cancer diagnosis of a dear friend of hers. This patient is now very upset because she is just now hearing the news from strangers (receptionists) and had no idea her friend had cancer. She made the statement "I wonder if you all talk about me when I am not in the office. Maybe I should switch physicians."

What is wrong with this scenario?

_____

_____

What can be done to correct the problem and ensure that each patient is treated with confidentiality?

_____

_____

SCENARIO #2

On Monday you receive a call from a lawyer requesting medical records to be sent to his office on your patient Mr. John Cramer. Your receptionist honors his request by sending the records. On Friday you receive a call from Mr. Cramer screaming in your ear that you sent the records to a lawyer that was not on his side (patient is plaintiff vs defendant) without his permission to do so.
Mr. Cramer states you have violated his trust and confidentiality, ruined his case, and he is now going to sue the physician.

What was wrong with this scenario?

_____

_____

_____

_____

Have a classmate role-play this one with you for completion of necessary forms.

What could have been done differently to avoid this from happening in the future and maintain patient confidentiality?

_____

_____

_____

_____

ACKNOWLDEDGMENT OF RECEIPT OF NOTICE OF

PRIVACY PRACTICES

I have been provided with a copy of your Notice of Privacy Practices, which contains a description of how my Personal Health Information (PHI) is used and shared.

_____   _____

Signature of Patient/Representative   Date

_____

Relationship to Patient

If unable to sign document, state reason:

_____

_____

_____

Authorization for Release of Medical Records

I, _____ (patient or legal guardian), give permission to

_____ to release my medical records to

_____.

I understand that my medical records include documentation about my health, diagnostic testing, and financial information.

_____   _____

Signature   Date

CONSENT TO THE USE AND DISCLOSURE OF HEALTH INFORMATION FOR TREATMENT, PAYMENT, OR HEALTH CARE OPERATIONS

Name _____

Birthdate _____ SS# _____

I understand that as part of my health care, this organization originates and maintains health records describing my health history, symptoms, examination and test results, diagnoses, treatment, and any plan for future treatment or care.

I understand that this information serves as
- A basis for care and treatment
- A way of health-care providers communicating with regard to my treatment and care
- Information that assists for services billed and a means by which third-party payers can verify that a service billed was actually provided
- A means for assessing care quality and review of the competence of health-care professionals.

I understand I have the right to
- Object to any of the above statements
- Request restrictions as to how my health information will be used
- Revoke this consent in writing, except to the extent that the organization has already taken action thereon.

I request the following restrictions to the use or disclosure of my health information.

_____

_____

_____

_____

_____ _____ _____
Signature: Patient/Legal Representative Date Witness

OFFICE USE ONLY:

Accepted
Denied

_____ _____ _____
Signature Title Date

Practicum 3. Professionalism

COMPETENCY

CAAHEP: 3. c. (2) (b) Perform within legal and ethical boundaries
ABHES: 1. (a) Project a positive attitude
            1. (d) Be cognizant of ethical boundaries
            1. (g) Evidence a responsible attitude
            1. (i) Conduct work within scope of education, training, and ability
            2. (p) Professional components
            2. (q) Allied health professions and credentialing
            5. (f) Maintain licenses and accreditation
            6. (e) Maintain liability coverage

SPECIFIC TASK

Using reference material such as your textbook and openly discussing these issues with your classmate and instructor, state on the enclosed form:

- How the medical assistant and the physician can apply legal and ethical standards in the workplace
- Display a positive and responsible attitude
- Work within your scope of practice
- Maintain licenses, accreditations, and liability coverage
- Spell correctly and write neatly

STANDARD PRECAUTIONS

NA

EQUIPMENT/SUPPLIES

Reference source (textbooks)
Black pen

STANDARD OF PERFORMANCE OF THE TASK

You may earn a maximum of 5 points for each competency regardless of the number of steps to be performed.

    EX: If you miss two steps and achieve all the rest then you have earned 3 points. More than five steps missed means that you have 0 points.

    Your instructor may choose not to assign points but check you off on a pass or fail status. Regardless, you may need to repeat the competency for successful completion.

    It is up to your instructor to determine the maximum number of tries before the competency has been met successfully in the time allotted.

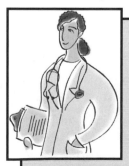

Make a Difference

There are many legal and ethical boundaries as a health-care practitioner. Projecting a positive and responsible attitude will assist you when dealing with ethical situations that could potentially cause liabilities to occur. Displaying professional components, working within your scope of training and becoming credentialed will earn you respect from the health-care community, and you will know that you have helped in making a difference where it really counts.

Student Name: _____ Date: _____

Time: Satisfactory   Unsatisfactory

Successful Completion: Yes   No

Grade/Points: _____   Pass   Fail

Need to Repeat: _____   Number of Attempts: 1   2   3

Instructor Comments: _____

_____

_____

CONDITIONS UNDER WHICH THE STUDENT IS EXPECTED TO PERFORM THE TASK

Follow Task/Performance Steps

	Task/Performance Step	S	U
1.	Student defines the difference between law and ethics.		
2.	Student demonstrates understanding of the medical assistant's scope of practice and limitations.		
3.	Student identifies the three penalties the physician may face in violation of ethical principles.		
4.	The student identifies three primary ethical standards that must be adhered to in the medical office.		
5.	Student identifies steps to be followed when addressing ethical dilemmas.		
6.	Student identifies elements of a teamwork approach between medical assistant and physician that enables each to perform within ethical boundaries.		
7.	Student actively participated with group discussion answering and defining the questions.		
8.	Student spells correctly and writes neatly.		
9.	Student answered all questions in writing.		

Key: Satisfactory = S; Unsatisfactory = U

SMART THINKING

1. **State the difference between law and ethics.**

_____

_____

_____

_____

2. Define the medical assistant's scope of practice and state limitations to the practice of medical assisting in your state, if any.

_____

_____

_____

_____

3. Name three penalties the physician may face in violation of ethical principles.

a. _____

_____

b. _____

_____

c. _____

_____

4. Name three primary ethical standards that must be adhered to in the medical office.

a. _____

_____

b. _____

_____

c. _____

_____

5. What steps can you follow when addressing ethical dilemmas?

a. _____

_____

b. _____

_____

c. _____

_____

6.   How can the medical assistant and the physician work together to perform within ethical boundaries?

a. _____

_____

b. _____

_____

c. _____

_____

7.   Name at least 10 attributes of the medical assistant that can help you portray a positive attitude.

a. _____

_____

b. _____

_____

c. _____

_____

d. _____

_____

e. _____

_____

f. _____

_____

g. _____

_____

h. _____

_____

i. _____

_____

j. _____

_____

8. State the two credentials that are accepted and widely known for medical assistants.

a. _____

_____

b. _____

_____

9. What do you believe is the number-one way you can show evidence of a responsible attitude?

_____

_____

_____

_____

GROUP DISCUSSION WITH CLASSMATES AND INSTRUCTOR

1. What type of accreditation does your institution (college) have?

_____

_____

_____

_____

2. What type of accreditation does your program have?

_____

_____

_____

3. Name just a few basic steps that must be done to maintain these accreditations?

_____

_____

_____

_____

4. Name several types of health-care practitioners' licenses and what they must do to maintain these credentials.

_____

_____

_____

_____

_____

5. What must you do to maintain your certification/registration once you have achieved your credentials?

_____

_____

_____

_____

6. Why is it important to maintain liability coverage?

_____

_____

_____

_____

7. As a medical assistant, how would you find this type of coverage?

_____

_____

_____

_____

Practicum 4. Legislative Issues

COMPETENCY

CAAHEP: 3. C. (2) (f) Demonstrate knowledge of federal and state health-care legislation and regulations

ABHES: 5. (e) Dispose of controlled substances in compliance with government regulations

5. (g) Monitor legislation related to current health-care issues and practices

SPECIFIC TASK

Research and state below several federal and state health-care legislative laws and regulations. Attach your findings below and discuss your research with your fellow classmates and instructor verbally. Spell correctly and demonstrate good writing skills.

STANDARD PRECAUTIONS

NA

EQUIPMENT/SUPPLIES

Black pen
Reference material (textbook)
Internet access or reference library

STANDARD OF PERFORMANCE OF THE TASK

You may earn a maximum of 5 points for each competency regardless of the number of steps to be performed.

EX: If you miss two steps and achieve all the rest then you have earned 3 points.

More than five steps missed means that you have 0 points.

Your instructor may choose not to assign points but check you off on a pass or fail status.

Regardless, you may need to repeat the competency for successful completion.

It is up to your instructor to determine the maximum number of tries before the competency has been met successfully in the time allotted.

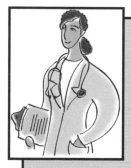

Make a Difference

Laws and regulations can affect us all. Acts are first introduced at the federal level. The acts are then voted on and passed by the United States Congress. Your state legislation develops statutes, and your local governing bodies create the ordinances. It is extremely important to understand and know your federal and state health-care legislation and regulations and abide by them.

Student Name: _____   Date: _____

Time: Satisfactory   Unsatisfactory

Successful Completion: Yes   No

Grade/Points: _____   Pass   Fail

Need to Repeat: _____   Number of Attempts: 1   2   3

Instructor Comments: _____

_____

_____

CONDITIONS UNDER WHICH THE STUDENT IS EXPECTED TO PERFORM THE TASK

Follow Task/Performance Steps

Task/Performance Step	S	U
1. Student answered all questions correctly.		
2. Student actively participated in the group discussion about the disposal of controlled substances.		
3. Student found recent health-care legislation and attached to page. Student shared this information with the other classmates verbally.		
4. Student spelled words correctly and demonstrated good writing skills.		

Key: Satisfactory = S; Unsatisfactory = U

SMART THINKING

1. **When was HIPAA first introduced into legislation and passed?**

_____

_____

_____

2. **What are the two primary purposes of HIPAA?**

_____

_____

_____

3. **What is one of the most extensive privacy rules?**

_____

_____

_____

4.   When were the final regulations regarding the privacy legislation sections of HIPAA published?

_____

_____

_____

5.   Name at least two forms, notices, or consents that were created and must be used with patients with regard to medical records and confidentiality as a result of HIPAA legislation.

_____

_____

6.   Who was the president that signed the Occupational Safety and Health Act (OSHA)?

_____

_____

7.   What is OSHA's main focus and accomplishment?

_____

_____

8.   Who enforces CLIA? Is it a law?

_____

_____

GROUP DISCUSSION WITH CLASSMATES AND INSTRUCTOR

1.   The Department of Justice established the Drug Enforcement Administration (DEA) in 1973. There are many regulations with regard to controlled substances.

State the ways in which controlled substances must be disposed of to maintain compliance with government regulations.

_____

_____

_____

_____

_____

_____

_____

2. Research and monitor a recent health-care legislative issue and share this information with the class/instructor. You can clip a newspaper article or print Internet research and attach to this page.

_____

_____

_____

_____

_____

_____

_____

_____

_____

_____

_____

_____

_____

Practicum 5. Office Policies

COMPETENCY

CAAHEP: 3. c. (3) (a) Explain general office policies
ABHES: 7. (a) Orient patients to office policies and procedures

SPECIFIC TASK

Using a computer, create a patient information form explaining that your office expects payment when services are rendered. Attach your brochure/information packet below.

STANDARD PRECAUTIONS

NA

EQUIPMENT/SUPPLIES

Reference source (textbook)
Black pen
Computer with editing capability

STANDARD OF PERFORMANCE OF THE TASK

You may earn a maximum of 5 points for each competency regardless of the number of steps to be performed.

EX: If you miss two steps and achieve all the rest then you have earned 3 points.

More than five steps missed means that you have 0 points.

Your instructor may choose not to assign points but check you off on a pass or fail status.

Regardless, you may need to repeat the competency for successful completion.

It is up to your instructor to determine the maximum number of tries before the competency has been met successfully in the time allotted.

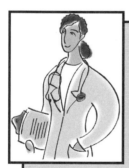

Make a Difference

Patients that are informed and understand your office policy before coming in as new patients are more likely to follow through with requests and treatment plans. Many offices create brochures that state various office policies and introduce the staff. These brochures are mailed with the new patient information forms to be completed ahead of scheduled appointments to help save time in the office and explain general office policy.

Student Name: _____   Date: _____

Time: Satisfactory   Unsatisfactory

Successful Completion: Yes   No

Grade/Points: _____   Pass   Fail

Need to Repeat: _____   Number of Attempts: 1   2   3

Instructor Comments: _____

_____

_____

CONDITIONS UNDER WHICH THE STUDENT IS EXPECTED TO PERFORM THE TASK

Follow Task/Performance Steps

Task/Performance Step	S	U
1. Assemble necessary supplies. *Having all supplies you will need together maximizes time management.*		
2. Student selects appropriate format to be used (i.e., Question and Answers, or list steps). *Correct format facilitates patient understanding.*		
3. Student creates patient information document describing the office policy of payment at time of services rendered. (refer to Database for office policy). *Written policies and documentation help clarify office procedure and patient responsibilities.*		
4. Student properly proofreads spelling and punctuation and reviews the contents of the document for all essential information. *Correct written communication reflects professionalism.*		
5. Student is able to explain the purpose and details of the policy when questioned by the patient. *Written information with verbal reinforcement should be required for complete patient understanding.*		

Key: Satisfactory = S; Unsatisfactory = U

Attach by stapling Information Document to this page.

Practicum 6. Patient Teaching

COMPETENCY

CAAHEP: 3. c. (3) (b) Instruct individuals according to their needs
          3. c. (3) (c) Provide instruction for health maintenance and disease prevention
ABHES: 2. (c) Adapt what is said to the recipient's level of comprehension
          2. (m) Adaptation for individualized needs
          7. (b) Instruct patients with special needs
          7. (c) Teach patients methods of health promotion and disease prevention

SPECIFIC TASK

Create a brochure or form letter using a word processor addressing the needs of a new mother and her newborn infant by providing instruction about the importance of and schedule for recommended immunizations to promote health maintenance and disease prevention. Create the document with a simple basic level of comprehension so that all individuals will understand.

The student will need to research and obtain information regarding immunizations using the textbook, library, or by calling a pediatric or family practice office.

Be sure to include Dr. Wright's name, address, and phone number on your form letter or brochure. This information can be found in the Database.

The student will attach the form letter/brochure to the page below.

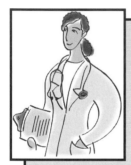

Make a Difference

Patients who are informed will most likely become their own advocate in health care. Informed patients can make wise health-care decisions with regard to treatment and options available. Information delivered to patients, keeping in mind their level of comprehension and individualized needs should assist them in understanding what is being stated. You are trained to understand medical terminology and language. The nonmedically trained individual does not always understand.

STANDARD PRECAUTIONS

NA

EQUIPMENT/SUPPLIES

Computer (word processor)
Printer/printer paper
Pen
Stapler
Attached form
Reference source for research information

STANDARD OF PERFORMANCE OF THE TASK

You may earn a maximum of 5 points for each competency regardless of the number of steps to be performed.

EX: If you miss two steps and achieve all the rest then you have earned 3 points.

More than five steps missed means that you have 0 points.

Your instructor may choose not to assign points but check you off on a pass or fail status.

Regardless, you may need to repeat the competency for successful completion.

It is up to your instructor to determine the maximum number of tries before the competency has been met successfully in the time allotted.

Student Name: _____   Date: _____

Time:	Satisfactory	Unsatisfactory
Successful Completion:	Yes	No
Grade/Points: _____	Pass	Fail

Need to Repeat: _____   Number of Attempts: 1   2   3

Instructor Comments: _____

_____

_____

CONDITIONS UNDER WHICH THE STUDENT IS EXPECTED TO PERFORM THE TASK

Follow Task/Performance Steps

Task/Performance Step	S	U
1. Student assembles equipment, supplies, and immunization information.		
2. Student turns on computer.		
3. Student selects word processing program to be used.		
4. Student creates a patient education form letter or brochure addressing the importance of immunizations and recommended schedule for a newborn infant.		
5. Student creates a title for the brochure/form letter.		
6. Student includes accurate information in the form letter.		
7. Student organizes the information and uses terms that are easily understandable and can be comprehended by the patient or primary care giver.		
8. Student edits text by pressing the arrow keys to move the cursor to the appropriate position to insert or delete characters.		
9. Student understands and uses computer commands to delete entire blocks of characters, including cutting and pasting of characters.		
10. Student uses spelling and grammar check to assist with the editing process.		
11. Student proofreads form for errors and accuracy.		
12. Student prints using the computer "print" command.		
13. Student saves document template by using the "save as" command to "C" drive (c:/), "A" drive (a:/), or CD-RW.		
14. Student instructs (role-play with another student) the mother of a newborn on the importance of immunizations and recommended immunization schedule using the brochure/form letter as a patient education tool.		
15. Student appropriately and accurately answers any questions the mother may have regarding immunizations.		
16. Student documents patient education given and mother's understanding of the instruction.		

Key: Satisfactory = S; Unsatisfactory = U

Patient Name: __Betsy Smith__

Progress Note:

Date: _____

_____

_____

_____

(Attach your brochure/form letter to this page)

Practicum 7. Working Within the Community

COMPETENCY

CAAHEP: 3. c. (3) (d) Identify community resources
ABHES: 3. (f) Locate resources and information for patients and employers
7. (b) Instruct patients with special needs

SPECIFIC TASK

Identify 10 community resources in your area and list the services that they provide, including:
- Contact person
- Telephone number
- When and where meetings/classes are held.
This information is helpful to patients and the employers that you may be employed by in the future.
Identify resources focusing on people with special needs. Complete your list on the attached information sheet.

STANDARD PRECAUTIONS

NA

EQUIPMENT/SUPPLIES

Resources: phonebook/newspaper/Web sites
Enclosed form
Pen

STANDARD OF PERFORMANCE OF THE TASK

You may earn a maximum of 5 points for each competency regardless of the number of steps to be performed.
EX: If you miss two steps and achieve all the rest then you have earned 3 points.
More than five steps missed means that you have 0 points.
Your instructor may choose not to assign points but check you off on a pass or fail status.
Regardless, you may need to repeat the competency for successful completion.
It is up to your instructor to determine the maximum number of tries before the competency has been met successfully in the time allotted.

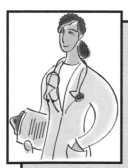

Make a Difference

Your office will not always be able to provide all the services that patients need and there are patients who require additional information that will assist them in accommodating any special needs. By knowing what services are offered in your community you will be able to assist the patient in many different ways, and your office will be viewed as helpful and courteous.

Student Name: _____   Date: _____

Time: Satisfactory   Unsatisfactory

Successful Completion: Yes   No

Grade/Points: _____   Pass   Fail

Need to Repeat: _____   Number of Attempts: 1   2   3

Instructor Comments: _____

_____

_____

CONDITIONS UNDER WHICH THE STUDENT IS EXPECTED TO PERFORM THE TASK

Follow Task/Performance Steps

Task/Performance Step	S	U
1. Student identifies 10 community resources on the page below.		
2. Student lists contact person and telephone number of each organization. *Providing contact information will save you and the patient time and aggravation.*		
3. Student identifies location where the meetings/classes are held. *This will assist the patient with transportation needs as many of the elderly ride buses or count on others to assist them.*		
4. Student lists dates and times when meetings/classes are held. *This assists the patient in being able to plan ahead and helps ensure that the patient will arrive on time.*		
5. Student list includes community resources that focus on individuals with special needs.		

Key: Satisfactory = S; Unsatisfactory = U

COMMUNITY RESOURCES/INFORMATION FOR PATIENTS/PHYSICIANS/EMPLOYERS

Facility	Location	Contact Person	Phone	Time Meetings Held
1.				
2.				

Facility	Location	Contact Person	Phone	Time Meetings Held
3.				
4.				
5.				
6.				
7.				
8.				
9.				
10.				

Practicum 8. Physician Management

COMPETENCY

CAAHEP: NA
ABHES: 3. (g) Manage physician's professional schedule and travel

SPECIFIC TASK

Your physician has been asked to speak at a national conference. He has asked that you take care of the travel arrangements. Create the physician's itinerary using the information and itinerary schedule provided below. You may hand write by using the attached form or create the schedule on the computer and attach to this competency by stapling.

There are four patients who will need to be rescheduled due to the physician's unexpected absence from the office. The patients are provided on the appointment schedule below. Role-play with a classmate and reschedule the patients using the proper telephone technique and appointment scheduling.

Schedule

Traveling to:	Orlando, FL
Airlines:	Quick Flights
Departs QC, FL:	10:05 AM – January 22, 20xx
Arrives, Orlando:	12:30 PM – January 22, 20xx
Hotel:	Florida's Finest Convention Center/Hotel
Rm. Confirm. No.:	XY359
Stay:	2 Nights
Presentation:	2:00 PM – January 23, 20xx Ballroom, 2nd Floor of the Plaza Family Practice Value and Quality: How Your Office Can Achieve Quality Care
Departs Orlando:	8:00 AM – January 24, 20xx
Arrives, QC, FL:	10:32 AM – January 24, 20xx (The physician has stated that he will see patients on the 24th starting at 12:00 PM)
Transportation:	Taxi
Special Requests:	Steak, Banquet Dinner – 7:00 PM Ballroom
Meeting a colleague:	Dr. Henegas at 7:00 PM on January 22, 20xx, for cocktails and dinner at the Perfect Lounge and Restaurant in the hotel lobby.
Reminders:	Doctor needs laptop computer and a CD with the presentation. Handouts have been mailed in advance and will be waiting at the concierge station.

STANDARD PRECAUTIONS

N/A

EQUIPMENT/SUPPLIES

Phone/appointment book/computer
Pen/preplanned schedule from physician

STANDARD OF PERFORMANCE OF THE TASK

You may earn a maximum of 5 points for each competency regardless of the number of steps to be performed.

EX: If you miss two steps and achieve all the rest then you have earned 3 points.

More than five steps missed means that you have 0 points.

Your instructor may choose not to assign points but check you off on a pass or fail status.

Regardless, you may need to repeat the competency for successful completion.

It is up to your instructor to determine the maximum number of tries before the competency has been met successfully in the time allotted.

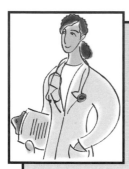

Make a Difference

Always make sure that the physician and the office have a copy of the itinerary and that you are aware of who the physician on-call is during your physician's absence. Always ask if there are any special considerations such as transportation or special food requests. Always have the Dr.'s beeper and cellular phone information in case your office needs to reach him/her.

Student Name: _____   Date: _____

Time: Satisfactory   Unsatisfactory

Successful Completion: Yes   No

Grade/Points: _____   Pass   Fail

Need to Repeat: _____   Number of Attempts: 1   2   3

Instructor Comments: _____

_____

_____

CONDITIONS UNDER WHICH THE STUDENT IS EXPECTED TO PERFORM THE TASK

Follow Task/Performance Steps

	Task/Performance Step	S	U
1.	Student confirms the physician's travel and special considerations.		
2.	Student creates the physician's itinerary with accuracy.		
3.	The student notes that the patients listed on January 23, Year, need to be rescheduled.		
4.	Student role-plays with a classmate and reschedules the patients on the day the physician will return after 12:00 PM.		
5.	Student demonstrated professionalism and scheduled the patients accurately.		

Key: Satisfactory = S; Unsatisfactory = U

PHYSICIAN ITINERARY

Date	Event/Time	Place	Who/What	Special Requests/Items

Date	Event/Time	Place	Who/What	Special Requests/Items

APPOINTMENT BOOK

Time	Date – 1/23		Date – 1/24		Notes:
7:00					
:30					
:45					
8:00	Quint, Patty – H&P	568-3810			
:15					
:30		.			
:45					
9:00	Kaine, Neil – Flu-F/U	562-8365	Doctor/Conference		
:15	Burke, Ethyl – P&P	321-7356			
:30					
:45					
10:00	Minton, Shelly – OV, Earache	562-7198			
:15					
:30					
:45					
11:00			Lunch		
:15					
:30					
:45					
12:00	Lunch				
:15					
:30			Cann, Antonio – BP Check	778-7329	
:45					
1:00					
:15					
:30					
:45					
2:00					
:15					
:30					
:45					
3:00					
:15					
:30					
:45					
4:00					
:15					
:30					

:45					
5:00					

(The physician stated he would see patients the day he returns.)

Practicum 9. Appointment Management

COMPETENCY

CAAHEP: 3. a. (1) (a) Schedule and manage appointments
 3. c. (4) (c) Utilize computer software to maintain office systems
 3. c. (1) (d) Demonstrate telephone technique
ABHES: 2. (e) Use proper telephone techniques
 2. (n) Application of electronic technology
 3. (c) Schedule and monitor appointments
 3. (d) Apply computer concepts for office procedures

SPECIFIC TASK

Schedule appointments using the appointment book attached and use your medical office computer software to schedule the same appointments after determining if and when a patient should be seen, keeping in mind the patient's needs and the physician's schedule and preferences. You will find this information in the Database at the front of this manual.

Following the procedural steps, make a determination and appointment within the time and accuracy specified by your instructor. Demonstrate telephone technique using a professional approach when scheduling appointments. Use the database and role-play with another student.

Following procedural steps outlined below, schedule and manage the incoming calls for appointment scheduling for 2 weeks using the patient list provided.

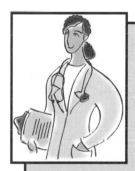

Make a Difference

Appointment books are considered legal documents and are subject to subpoena. Write or print clearly and make corrections neatly when entering appointments manually. Do not erase missed appointments. Put a line through the patient's name so it is still legible and make a notation next to patient's name indicating the status of the appointment (e.g., canceled, missed, or rescheduled). Never delete a patient's name from the computer schedule. Put R/S (Rescheduled) or NS (No-show) or CX (Cancelled) next to the patient name. Make sure the information is also noted in the patient chart.

STANDARD PRECAUTIONS

NA

EQUIPMENT/SUPPLIES

Database/scheduling guidelines
Appointment book/pages
Appointment card
Pen
Telephone
Computer with medical appointment software

STANDARD OF PERFORMANCE OF THE TASK

You may earn a maximum of 5 points for each competency regardless of the number of steps to be performed.

EX: If you miss two steps and achieve all the rest then you have earned 3 points.

More than five steps missed means that you have 0 points.

Your instructor may choose not to assign points but check you off on a pass or fail status.

Regardless, you may need to repeat the competency for successful completion.

It is up to your instructor to determine the maximum number of tries before the competency has been met successfully in the time allotted.

Student Name: _____   Date: _____

Time:	Satisfactory	Unsatisfactory
Successful Completion:	Yes	No
Grade/Points: _____	Pass	Fail
Need to Repeat: _____	Number of Attempts: 1 2 3	

Instructor Comments: _____

_____

_____

CONDITIONS UNDER WHICH THE STUDENT IS EXPECTED TO PERFORM THE TASK

Follow Task/Performance Steps

Task/Performance Step	S	U
1. Create the Matrix for the week of April 1–5 for Dr. Wright using the attached appointment sheets and your computer software. Refer to the database for office hours, and block out unavailable times according to physician's preference. *Physician is unable to see patients during lunch, meetings, hospital rounds, and procedures/surgery. This prevents you from having to cancel or reschedule a patient in the future.*		
2. Each student role-plays, pretending to be one of the patients from the list with another student answering the telephone using courtesy and a positive attitude. *Initial impressions reflect a smile in your voice and professionalism of the entire office.*		
3. Refer to database and schedule office appointments in the appointment book provided and on the computer. Include the patient's phone number, reason for visit, whether patient is established (EP) or new (NP). *New patients require more time than established patients.*		
4. Student uses proper telephone protocol and states greeting, time of day, name of establishment, medical assistant's name, "how can I help you?" and nature of the call. *Shows professionalism and a good first impression.*		
5. Student properly extracts pertinent information from the caller. *Pertinent information includes the following:* • *Patient's name in full* • *Source of referral* • *DOB* • *New or established patient* • *Daytime phone number* • *Reason for call (appointment)* • *Complete address* • *Insurance coverage*		
6. Referring to the database provided, student identifies patient Ken Slate's reason for visit. Student then correctly determines the need for a same-day appointment. *Urgency of appointments may be determined by severity of the caller's concern.*		
7. Student offers appropriate choice of days and times for appointment. *Patients feel more in control if given a choice.*		
8. Student enters the patient's name, phone number, reason for visit and NP or EP in the appointment book and in the computer next to the mutually agreeable time. *Consider time allotment for common office procedures in Database.*		

9. Student establishes if patient is expected to pay a co-pay or payment for services rendered at time of visit. *Patients should be informed of office policy regarding financial arrangements before the actual visit.*		
10. Student explains financial arrangement policy of office and reminds patient to bring insurance card at time of visit. *This helps to defray collection costs in the future.*		
11. Student offers caller directions to the office. *Clear directions help alleviate patient anxiety regarding the location of office.*		
12. Student repeats to patient the date and time of appointment. *Repeating allows for patient verification.*		
13. Student follows office policy regarding sending of appointment cards and/or new patient forms in advance. *Forms sent in advance allow the patient to complete at their convenience, allowing for better office time management and advance questions from the patient.*		
14. Student closes telephone interaction addressing caller cordially.		
WALK-IN PATIENT		
15. Student acknowledges patient (role-play with classmate) promptly, greets patient in friendly, professional manner, introduces self, and welcomes patient and/or family to the office. *You are the first impression of the office and the physician.*		
16. Student asks appropriate questions as defined in steps #2 and #5. *Consider patient confidentiality if other patients are within hearing distance. HIPAA compliance.*		
17. Follow steps #6 through #12. *Asking the patient to clarify assists in your both having the same understanding.*		
18. Student completes appointment card attached with all the necessary information. Ask the patient if there are any questions and if they understand. *Complete all information, write neatly, use AM/PM for clarity.*		
19. Student gives appointment card to patient verifying day, date, and time of appointment and closes conversation cordially.		

Key: Satisfactory = S; Unsatisfactory = U

PATIENTS REQUIRING APPOINTMENTS*

a. Sandra Backer – sore throat
b. Dan Olstine – H&P
c. Kris Hardee – fever
d. Patrice Roc – swollen foot
e. Ken Slate – difficulty voiding
f. Debbie Verisso – BP follow-up
g. Darcee Rooso – cough/cold
h. Lindy Schaffer – high fever

i. Marcus Plan – headache x3d
j. Antonio Cann – cast removal
k. Mary Manygrats – chest pain
l. Patty Quint – flu injection
m. Neil Kaine – suture removal
n. Earnest Swain – fever/irritable
o. Dillon Ocerby – well-child visit/immunization

*Don't forget to complete the appointment cards for those patients who will be returning to your clinic. You should have cards for all walk-in patients.

SMART THINKING

1. What information is important to obtain when the pharmacist calls and is requesting a patient medication refill?

_____

_____

_____

2. Before placing a caller on hold, what important information should be obtained first?

_____

_____

_____

_____

3. What is good telephone technique when dealing with the angry caller?

_____

_____

_____

_____

4. Why is it important to create the Matrix first?

_____

_____

_____

_____

5. Using 11:00 AM Eastern Time, what time is it if a call is placed to a physician who is located in Pacific Time? What time is it if the call was placed to Mountain time? What time is it if the call was placed to Central time?

_____

_____

_____

_____

6. What time is 1400 hours?

_____

APPOINTMENT BOOK

Time	Date – 4/1	Date – 4/2	Date – 4/3	Date – 4/4	Date – 4/5
7:00					
:15					
:30					
:45					
8:00					
:15					
:30					
:45					
9:00					
:15					
:30					
:45					
10:00					
:15					
:30					
:45					
11:00					
:15					
:30					
:45					
12:00					
:15					
:30					
:45					
1:00					
:15					
:30					
:45					
2:00					
:15					
:30					
:45					
3:00					
:15					
:30					
:45					
4:00					
:15					
:30					
:45					
5:00					

APPOINTMENT BOOK

Time	Date – 4/8	Date – 4/8	Date – 4/10	Date – 4/11	Date – 4/12
7:00					
:15					
:30					
:45					
8:00					
:15					
:30					
:45					
9:00					
:15					
:30					
:45					
10:00					
:15					
:30					
:45					
11:00					
:15					
:30					
:45					
12:00					
:15					
:30					
:45					
1:00					
:15					
:30					
:45					
2:00					
:15					
:30					
:45					
3:00					
:15					
:30					
:45					
4:00					
:15					
:30					
:45					
5:00					

APPOINTMENT CARDS

Dr. Franklin Pierce Wright, Family Practice
2310 Wright Way
Melbourne, FL 32904

Appointment for:

M_____

Month _____ Date _____

Day _____

Time _____ AM/PM

Dr. Franklin Pierce Wright, Family Practice
2310 Wright Way
Melbourne, FL 32904

Appointment for:

M_____

Month _____ Date _____

Day _____

Time _____ AM/PM

Dr. Franklin Pierce Wright, Family Practice
2310 Wright Way
Melbourne, FL 32904

Appointment for:

M_____

Month _____ Date _____

Day _____

Time _____ AM/PM

Dr. Franklin Pierce Wright, Family Practice
2310 Wright Way
Melbourne, FL 32904

Appointment for:

M_____

Month _____ Date _____

Day _____

Time _____ AM/PM

Dr. Franklin Pierce Wright, Family Practice
2310 Wright Way
Melbourne, FL 32904

Appointment for:

M_____

Month _____ Date _____

Day _____

Time _____ AM/PM

Dr. Franklin Pierce Wright, Family Practice
2310 Wright Way
Melbourne, FL 32904

Appointment for:

M_____

Month _____ Date _____

Day _____

Time _____ AM/PM

Dr. Franklin Pierce Wright, Family Practice
2310 Wright Way
Melbourne, FL 32904

Appointment for:

M_____

Month _____ Date _____

Day _____

Time _____ AM/PM

Dr. Franklin Pierce Wright, Family Practice
2310 Wright Way
Melbourne, FL 32904

Appointment for:

M_____

Month _____ Date _____

Day _____

Time _____ AM/PM

Practicum 10. Admissions

COMPETENCY

CAAHEP: 3. a. (1) (b) Schedule inpatient and outpatient admissions and procedures
         3. a. (3) (a) Apply managed care policies and procedures
ABHES: 3. (h) Schedule inpatient and outpatient admissions
         3. (u) Apply managed care policies and procedures
         3. (v) Obtain managed care referrals and precertification

SPECIFIC TASK

In the time specified by the instructor, schedule a patient following the steps below for an inpatient and an outpatient procedure using the attached physician order.

Obtain a managed care referral for the patient Darcee Rooso as needed and obtain precertification for the patient Sandy Backer from the insurance carrier for the procedure(s) and/or admission as ordered by the physician. Confirm and give all required instructions to the patient. Document all that was accomplished in the provided space. Patient insurance information is found in the Data Base.

STANDARD PRECAUTIONS

NA

EQUIPMENT/SUPPLIES

Telephone/pen/tablet
Physician's orders/referral form
Patient record
Patient's insurance information
Name, address, and telephone number of referral facility
Special preparation instructions for patient

STANDARD OF PERFORMANCE OF THE TASK

You may earn a maximum of 5 points for each competency regardless of the number of steps to be performed.
EX: If you miss two steps and achieve all the rest then you have earned 3 points.
More than five steps missed means that you have 0 points.
Your instructor may choose not to assign points but check you off on a pass or fail status. Regardless, you may need to repeat the competency for successful completion.
It is up to your instructor to determine the maximum number of tries before the competency has been met successfully in the time allotted.

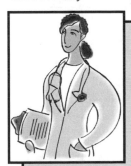

Make a Difference

HIPAA demands you maintain patient confidentiality. When scheduling or addressing patient concerns by phone it is important that you frequently check your immediate surroundings to ensure that no one has approached the front office area and is listening to the conversation. Remember, any type of patient information is confidential!

Student Name: _____   Date: _____

Time: Satisfactory   Unsatisfactory

Successful Completion: Yes   No

Grade/Points: _____   Pass   Fail

Need to Repeat: _____   Number of Attempts: 1   2   3

Instructor Comments: _____

_____

_____

CONDITIONS UNDER WHICH THE STUDENT IS EXPECTED TO PERFORM THE TASK

Follow Task/Performance Steps

Task/Performance Step	S	U
OUTPATIENT PROCEDURE AND MANAGED CARE REFERRAL		
1. Student obtains a written order from the physician for the outpatient procedure to be done for the patient Darcee Rooso. *Precise instructions from the physician will avoid misunderstandings and medical errors.*		
2. Student obtains referral from the patient's insurance carrier and documents on the referral form. Role-play by phone with another student. *Obtaining referrals and precertification numbers from a patient's insurance carrier helps to ensure payment for services rendered.*		
3. Student determines patient's availability. A classmate will role-play the patient. *This avoids scheduling conflicts and involves the patient.*		
4. Student organizes necessary scheduling information on a scratch pad before telephoning referral facility. *Necessary scheduling information includes patient's name, telephone number, age, birth date, and insurance carrier. You should also obtain the name and telephone number of referring facility, designated procedure, desired date, and special physician instructions for patient and/or facility.*		
5. Student places calls to both outpatient and referral facilities and states specifics required by physician. Student reports any referral/precertification numbers to the appropriate facilities. *Proper telephone etiquette and organization of scheduling information demonstrates professionalism and professional courtesy.*		
6. Student establishes a date and time for the outpatient procedure and the referral appointment. *Writing this information down will ensure accuracy.*		
7. Student obtains any special instructions for the procedure from the outpatient or referral facility to give to the patient. *Instructions in writing will help the patient to remember important steps, location, and times.*		

8.	Student notifies Darcee Rooso of the arrangements, including name, address, and telephone number of the referral facility, date and time of procedure, and any special instructions. *Good patient education helps the patient to prepare for and understand the procedure.*		
9.	Student requests patient to repeat instructions for verification. *Eliminates miscommunications and helps ensure patient understanding.*		
10.	Student documents arrangements in the progress note and any referral numbers on the patient's medical record. *If it wasn't documented, it wasn't done!*		
INPATIENT ADMISSION AND PRECERTIFICATION:			
11.	Student notes physician's order for Sandra Backer to be admitted to hospital. *Patients can only be admitted and treated with a physician's order.*		
12.	Student instructs/assists patient (Sandra Backer) for an inpatient admission following steps 1-11 as applicable for precertification number. *Without precertification, hospital stays and procedures are not covered.*		
13.	Student instructs patient to complete preadmission labs and forms before admission. *Tasks done ahead of time will help ease the patient's anxiety.*		
14.	Give patient all information regarding admission to hospital. Document. *Information given to the patient should include name, address, telephone number, and directions to the hospital if needed. Other information sent with patient should reflect physician protocol. (i.e., admitting orders, H&P, labs to be performed before any surgery, and/or results of diagnostic tests). Information can be faxed, telephoned, or sent with patient. Be sure to follow HIPAA regulations.*		

Key: Satisfactory = S; Unsatisfactory = U

PHYSICIAN'S ORDERS

Dr. Franklin Pierce Wright, Family Practice
2310 Wright Way
Melbourne, FL 32904
Telephone (904) 565-3200

Patient: Darcee Rooso

Date of birth (DOB): 12/23/47

Arthroscopy of the left knee. Discontinue the prescribed Aspirin for 3 days before the outpatient surgery. Patient is to be seen in follow-up 3 days after the procedure.

Refer this patient to Miracle Rehabilitation for therapy to left knee post arthroscopy.

Appointment should be made in advance so patient can begin therapy following

procedure and have ortho device ready to be placed and fitted.

Procedure Time: 60 minutes

Preop Laboratory: CBC

Diagnosis: Torn Ligament

Scratch Pad (For organizing patient information and times):

_____

_____

_____

_____

REFERRAL FORM

Dr. Franklin Pierce Wright, Family Practice
2310 Wright Way
Melbourne, FL 32904
Telephone (904) 565-3200

PATIENT NAME _____

AGE _____   DOB _____

GENDER _____

INSURANCE CARRIER _____   GROUP # _____

ID# _____   REFERRAL # _____

REFERRED TO _____

ADDRESS _____

TELEPHONE _____

APPOINTMENT DATE _____

REFERRAL REASON _____

Progress Note – Documentation

Patient <u>Darcee Rooso</u>   Date _____

DOB _____   Allergies _____

_____

_____

_____

_____

_____

_____

PRECERTIFICATION/VERIFICATION FOR ADMISSION TO HOSPITAL

PATIENT NAME ___Sandra Backer_____

AGE _____ DOB _____

GENDER _____

INSURANCE CARRIER _____ GROUP # _____

ID# _____ Precert # _____

REFERRED BY _____

FACILITY ADDRESS _____

TELEPHONE _____

DATE OF ADMISSION _____

DIAGNOSIS _____

LENGTH OF STAY CERTIFIED _____

SURGERY/PROCEDURES _____

CO-PAY/% AMOUNT TO PATIENT _____

Progress Note – Documentation

Patient ___Sandra Backer_____ Date _____

DOB _____ Allergies _____

_____

_____

_____

_____

_____

_____

_____

Practicum 11. Medical Records

COMPETENCY

CAAHEP: 3. a. (1) (c) Organize a patient's medical record
3. a. (1) (d) File medical records
3. c. (2) (c) Establish and maintain the medical record
ABHES: 3. (b) Prepare and maintain medical records
3. (i) File medical records

SPECIFIC TASK

Assemble and organize a patient's medical record using one name from the list of patient names we have supplied for you in the next page or use your name so you can continue to use the chart (medical record) throughout your course. Organize the medical record following the procedural steps using both the chronological sectional method and the problem-oriented medical record method. Include the new patient information sheet, history and physical form, signature on file form, progress notes, diagnostic and laboratory results, consultation reports, past medical record, correspondence related to patient care, prescription record, and insurance forms. Your instructor may provide a variety of forms not listed here.

Using the patient/medical records listed below, file the attached medical records using the alphabetical filing approach.

EQUIPMENT/SUPPLIES

Patient names/student names
Folder
Medical record forms
Black pen
Labels – letters, year, medical alert (optional)
Color-coded alphabetical tabs
File cabinet (optional)
Attached list of patient medical records for filing

STANDARD OF PERFORMANCE OF THE TASK

You may earn a maximum of 5 points for each competency regardless of the number of steps to be performed.

EX: If you miss two steps and achieve all the rest then you have earned 3 points.
More than five steps missed means that you have 0 points.
Your instructor may choose not to assign points but check you off on a pass or fail status.
Regardless, you may need to repeat the competency for successful completion.
It is up to your instructor to determine the maximum number of tries before the competency has been met successfully in the time allotted.

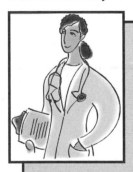

Make a Difference

Medical records are considered legal documents. Patient confidentiality must be maintained (HIPAA). Medical records must be kept in a secure area away from other patients and unauthorized personnel. When working with computerized records, caution must be taken to maintain the security of the records. Make sure that log-in passwords and codes are changed frequently and screens are in a direction that can only be seen by you. All documents are filed in Reverse Chronological Order.

Student Name: _____ Date: _____

Time: Satisfactory   Unsatisfactory

Successful Completion: Yes   No

Grade/Points: _____   Pass   Fail

Need to Repeat: _____   Number of Attempts: 1   2   3

Instructor Comments: _____

_____

_____

CONDITIONS UNDER WHICH THE STUDENT IS EXPECTED TO PERFORM THE TASK

Follow Task/Performance Steps

Task/Performance Step	S	U
1. Student assembles supplies. *A professional is always prepared.*		
2. Student obtains a label and writes the patient's full name for alphabetical filing. (Ex: Jonas, Thomas T.)		
3. Student color-codes the medical record by using a five-color–coding system with the first two letters of the last name and the first letter of the first name. (Your instructor may deviate from this plan if color labels are not available.) *The color-coded system is the most widely used for ease of retrieval of the chart (medical record).*		
4. Student places the patient label along the tabbed (indented lines) edge of the folder.		
5. Student places (or writes) a year label along the tabbed edge of the folder. *This identifies the year the patient first visited the practice and makes purging charts much easier. This label is changed each time the patient comes in the following new year.*		
6. Student organizes all the forms in the medical record including the problem or source-oriented record. *Types of records used and the organization will be determined by the physician/clinic protocol and will vary greatly from site to site and across the nation.*		
7. Student legibly writes patient's name on all forms to be included in the medical record. *Medical records are legal documents and must reflect patient identification on each form.*		
8. Role-play with a fellow classmate and complete the required patient information sheet and place it in the left front cover of the file. You may make up personal and health information or use the Database. Student also obtains "Signature on File" and signatures for any HIPAA consents. *After the patient has completed this form, double-check to make sure there are no blanks or inaccurate information. Accurate insurance information will assist with the insurance billing and collections. Always make a copy of the patient's insurance card, front and back, and store in the record.*		

9.	Role-plays and completes the patient history form and reviews it for completeness and accuracy. *Items incorrectly circled or misspelled can cause medical errors.*		
10.	Add labels to the chart that depict medical alerts, e.g., allergies, insurance, advanced directives. *HIPAA says this information can no longer be displayed on the outside of the chart because this is private patient information.*		
11.	Correctly file the charts we have attached by names only. Your instructor may choose to have you file your newly assembled files. *Correct filing technique facilitates quick retrieval of records.*		

Key: Satisfactory = S; Unsatisfactory = U

SMART THINKING

Number charts in alphabetical order.

LIST OF PATIENT MEDICAL RECORDS FOR FILING

	Last Name	First Name	MI
_____	Smith	John	
_____	Smith	Lori	
_____	Smith	John	T.
_____	Cooper	Smith	
_____	McBride	Debbie	
_____	McDonald	Sally	
_____	McBride	Deborah	
_____	MacBride	Patty	
_____	Jones	Kris	
_____	Jones	Petunia	J.
_____	Jones	Peter	J., Jr.

Practicum 12. Terminating Medical Treatment

COMPETENCY

CAAHEP: NA
ABHES: 5. (d) Follow established policy in initiating or terminating medical treatment

SPECIFIC TASK

In the time specified by your instructor, write a letter to a patient who will not follow through with the physician's medical advice or recommended treatment plan. Follow proper protocol with regard to terminating a patient. Use the patient name and information below and the example letter that has been provided.

Patient's Name: Ima Notgoingtodoit
40 Won't Comply Ave.
QC, FL 24590
Condition: Needs Angioplasty or patient will die

STANDARD PRECAUTIONS

NA

EQUIPMENT/SUPPLIES

Computer/editing capability
Paper

STANDARD OF PERFORMANCE OF THE TASK

You may earn a maximum of 5 points for each competency regardless of the number of steps to be performed.

EX: If you miss two steps and achieve all the rest then you have earned 3 points.
More than five steps missed means that you have 0 points.
Your instructor may choose not to assign points but check you off on a pass or fail status.
Regardless, you may need to repeat the competency for successful completion.
It is up to your instructor to determine the maximum number of tries before the competency has been met successfully in the time allotted.

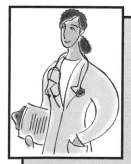

Make a Difference

A physician may not discontinue treatment of a patient as long as treatment is medically necessary. Termination of a patient is considered risk management and must be done according to the law. The only way a patient can be terminated is if a reasonable amount of time is given to the patient to find another physician. Until that time, the physician must see and treat the patient. Many times physicians will terminate the patient if the patient is not following prescribed advice or treatment plans that are critical to the patient's well-being.

Student Name: _____   Date: _____

Time: Satisfactory   Unsatisfactory

Successful Completion: Yes   No

Grade/Points: _____   Pass   Fail

Need to Repeat: _____   Number of Attempts: 1   2   3

Instructor Comments: _____

_____

_____

CONDITIONS UNDER WHICH THE STUDENT IS EXPECTED TO PERFORM THE TASK

Follow Task/Performance Steps

Task/Performance Step	S	U
1. Student demonstrates understanding of patient termination laws.		
2. Student writes letter of "Withdrawal From a Case."		
3. Student checks letter for accuracy and all necessary information.		
4. Student has physician (instructor) sign the letter and documents in the medical record what action was taken.		

Key: Satisfactory = S; Unsatisfactory = U

EXAMPLE LETTER

Letter of Withdrawal From a Case

Date

Name/Address

Dear Patient,

Recently, it has come to my attention that you have decided not to follow my medical advice or recommended treatment plan. I have encouraged you to also seek a second opinion so that you may understand the serious nature of your illness.

At this time, I find it necessary to inform you that I am withdrawing from further professional attendance on you for the above reason.

You require immediate medical attention and treatment; therefore, I recommend that you immediately seek the care of another physician.

I will allow you a reasonable time allotment of 30 days in which to seek further medical care from another physician. Until that time, I will continue to be your attending physician. After 30 days from receipt of this letter, I will no longer be able to provide you any medical services or advice.

My office would be happy to recommend other competent physicians, or you may choose to find one on your own.

Your medical condition is serious, so please don't delay. With your written permission, this office will send your medical record containing the diagnosis and treatment you have already received to the physician of your choice.

Very truly yours,

Signature

Remember: If it wasn't documented, it wasn't done.

PROGRESS NOTE:

_____

_____

_____

_____

_____

_____

_____

Attach your letter to this page by stapling.

Practicum 13. Medical Transcription

COMPETENCY

CAAHEP: NA
ABHES: 3. (e) Perform medical transcriptions

SPECIFIC TASK

Following the procedural steps below, transcribe an Operative Report and a Progress Report with 100% accuracy in a final draft, within the time specified by the instructor.

An example of an Operative Report has been provided for you. Do not copy this example. Your instructor will provide you with the necessary tapes and documents to type. Attach your transcribed reports below by stapling to the page.

STANDARD PRECAUTIONS

NA

EQUIPMENT/SUPPLIES

Dictation machine
Dictation cassette tape
Word processor or typewriter
Paper/printer
Dictionary/reference books

STANDARD OF PERFORMANCE OF THE TASK

You may earn a maximum of 5 points for each competency regardless of the number of steps to be performed.

EX: If you miss two steps and achieve all the rest then you have earned 3 points.

More than five steps missed means that you have 0 points.

Your instructor may choose not to assign points but check you off on a pass or fail status. Regardless, you may need to repeat the competency for successful completion.

It is up to your instructor to determine the maximum number of tries before the competency has been met successfully in the time allotted.

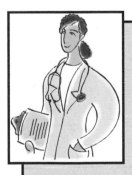

Make a Difference

Transcribing dictation is one of the administrative functions that a medical assistant may be required to perform. Transcription can be performed from a dictation machine or from handwritten notes. Typing speed, accuracy, and knowledge of medical terms are essential to perform this task with speed and competence. Many medical assistants choose to perform transcription at home to supplement their income. Productivity will depend on how quickly and accurately you type. The more you type the more you are paid!

Student Name: _____   Date: _____

Time: Satisfactory   Unsatisfactory

Successful Completion: Yes   No

Grade/Points: _____   Pass   Fail

Need to Repeat: _____   Number of Attempts: 1   2   3

Instructor Comments: _____

_____

_____

CONDITIONS UNDER WHICH THE STUDENT IS EXPECTED TO PERFORM THE TASK

Follow Task/Performance Steps

Task/Performance Step	S	U
1. Student assembles equipment and supplies.		
2. Student turns on dictation machine.		
3. Student turns on word processor, typewriter, or computer.		
4. Student inserts paper into word processor, typewriter, or printer.		
5. Student sets volume, tone, speed, and controls on dictation machine. *Setting controls according to your needs allows for accurate comprehension of dictation.*		
6. Student adjusts volume, tone, speed, and controls as needed for clarity of dictation. *Adjusting controls as needed enhances clarity.*		
7. Student types a draft of dictated operative report using correct format (see example) and leaves blanks where certain words are in question.		
8. Student consults reference books as needed for correct word identification. *Many medical terms have similar pronunciations. It is important to select the correct word as dictated by the physician.*		
9. Student proofreads the draft.		
10. Student consults dictionary and reference books for correct word spelling. *Using reference books helps ensure the correct word is selected and spelled correctly and ensures accuracy of the dictation.*		
11. Student corrects errors and fills in blanks.		
12. Student types (typewriter) or saves and prints (word processor or computer) the final copy.		
13. Student types a dictated progress report and follows steps 6–12.		
14. Student shuts down machines.		
15. Student obtains physician's signature (instructor) on final copy of the operative report and progress report. *Transcribed reports are not considered final until signed by the physician (Risk Management).*		
16. Student attaches files below. *The reports would then be placed in the patient medical record.*		

Key: Satisfactory = S; Unsatisfactory = U

EXAMPLE

OPERATIVE REPORT

Name: Tie Priter   #190456   Surgery 200-A

Date of Surgery :   September 22, Year

Preoperative Diagnosis: Hematuria, transitional cell carcinoma of the bladder with radiation cystitis and proctitis.

Postoperative Diagnosis: Bleeding from prostatic bed.

Procedure: TUR, biopsy, and fulguration of prostatic bed.

Procedure: With patient in the dorsal lithotomy position after satisfactory spinal anesthesia, a 28 Storz rectoscope was introduced into the prostate

Attach transcription to this page:

1. **Operative report**
2. **Progress report**

Practicum 14. Petty Cash

COMPETENCY

CAAHEP: NA
ABHES: 3. (o) Establish and maintain a petty cash fund

SPECIFIC TASK

Establish a petty cash fund. Prepare and record petty cash vouchers with 100% accuracy. Maintain an accurate record of expenditures for a specified time and replenish fund as necessary.

STANDARD PRECAUTIONS

NA

EQUIPMENT/SUPPLIES

Pen
Check in the amount of $50.00 to initiate fund
Petty cash record forms
Petty cash vouchers
Disbursement journal

STANDARD OF PERFORMANCE OF THE TASK

You may earn a maximum of 5 points for each competency regardless of the number of steps to be performed.
    EX: If you miss two steps and achieve all the rest then you have earned 3 points.
    More than five steps missed means that you have 0 points.
    Your instructor may choose not to assign points but check you off on a pass or fail status.
Regardless, you may need to repeat the competency for successful completion.
    It is up to your instructor to determine the maximum number of tries before the competency has been met successfully in the time allotted.

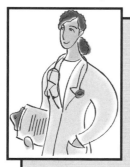

Make a Difference

Petty cash funds are established to help with minor office costs such as postage and miscellaneous spending. The main reason for a petty cash fund and voucher system is because change can be made for the patient who pays with cash. Maintaining this fund should be the responsibility of one individual so there are not too many "hands in the pot."

Student Name: _____   Date: _____

Time: Satisfactory   Unsatisfactory

Successful Completion: Yes   No

Grade/Points: _____   Pass   Fail

Need to Repeat: _____   Number of Attempts: 1   2   3

Instructor Comments: _____

_____

_____

CONDITIONS UNDER WHICH THE STUDENT IS EXPECTED TO PERFORM THE TASK

Follow Task/Performance Steps

Task/Performance Step	S	U
1. Student determines amount needed in petty cash fund. *Most offices will begin with $50.00 in various bills.*		
2. Student records beginning balance in petty cash record. *Your beginning balance would be $50.00.*		
3. Student posts initial check for petty cash fund to disbursement journal. *All checks paid should be recorded in the disbursement journal.*		
4. Student prepares a voucher for expenditures shown. *This allows you to keep track of who receives the money and for what.*		
5. Student records expenditures shown in the petty cash record and calculates the new balance. *This allows you to keep track of the balance so you know when the account needs to be replenished.*		
6. Student totals expense column on petty cash record. *This shows your new total or what is left in the account.*		
7. Student posts total of expense column on the petty cash record to the disbursement journal as a debit.		
8. Student records unused petty cash in the credit column of the disbursement journal.		
9. Student records funds needed to replenish petty cash on the petty cash record and disbursement journal.		

Key: Satisfactory = S; Unsatisfactory = U

Dr. Franklin Pierce Wright , Family Practice 9412
2310 Wright Way
Melbourne, FL 32904   Date **May 1,**
2000 _____

Pay to the
Order of _____**Cash**_____ $ _____50.00_____

_____**Fifty and no 00/00**__ Dollars

Community Bank

For ____**Petty cash fund**____

Using the following list of expenditures, document on the vouchers and petty cash record as follows:

5-1-00	Fund established	$50.00	Jennifer Lope/Secretary
5-3-00	Postage due	$6.00	Jennifer Lope, RMA
5-8-00	Parking fee	$5.00	Dr. Wright
5-12-00	Delivery charge	$3.85	Barbara Kendall, CMA
5-20-00	Stationery supplies	$8.55	Jennifer Lope

PETTY CASH RECORD

No.	Date	Description	Amount	Office Exp.	Misc.	Balance

PETTY CASH VOUCHERS

Amount $_____ No. _____	Amount $_____ No. _____
Received of Petty Cash	Received of Petty Cash
For_____	For_____
Charge to_____	Charge to_____
Approved by Received by	Approved by Received by
_____ _____	_____ _____
Amount $_____ No. _____	Amount $_____ No. _____
Received of Petty Cash	Received of Petty Cash
For_____	For_____
Charge to_____	Charge to_____
Approved by Received by	Approved by Received by
_____ _____	_____ _____
Amount $_____ No. _____	Amount $_____ No. _____
Received of Petty Cash	Received of Petty Cash
For_____	For_____
Charge to_____	Charge to_____
Approved by Received by	Approved by Received by
_____ _____	_____ _____

Disbursement Journal:

Date	Account Title and Explanation	Debit	Credit

Practicum 15. Bank Transactions

COMPETENCY

CAAHEP: 3. a. (2) (a) Prepare a bank deposit
ABHES: 3. (a) Perform basic secretarial skills
           3. (j) Prepare a bank statement
           3. (k) Reconcile a bank statement
           8. (e) Maintain records for accounting and banking purposes

SPECIFIC TASK

Performing bank deposits, preparing and reconciling bank statements, and maintaining these records are a part of the basic tasks that a secretary or front office personnel would perform.

- Prepare a bank deposit slip for depositing currency and checks for the day's receipts using the attached.
- Endorse the checks provided. Include "for deposit only," physician signature or stamp, and account number on the back of the check.
- Prepare and maintain your bank statement by checking off the listed checks cleared.
- Reconcile (confirming bank statement and checkbook balance are in agreement) a bank statement. Use the bank reconciliation worksheet provided.

STANDARD PRECAUTIONS

N/A

EQUIPMENT/SUPPLIES

Calculator
Pen/pencil
Attached checks for endorsement
Deposit slip
Deposit envelope
Attached bank reconciliation form/statement

STANDARD OF PERFORMANCE OF THE TASK

You may earn a maximum of 5 points for each competency regardless of the number of steps to be performed.
　　EX: If you miss two steps and achieve all the rest then you have earned 3 points.
　　More than five steps missed means that you have 0 points.
　　Your instructor may choose not to assign points but check you off on a pass or fail status.
Regardless, you may need to repeat the competency for successful completion.
　　It is up to your instructor to determine the maximum number of tries before the competency has been met successfully in the time allotted.

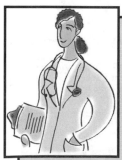

Make a Difference

Financial records are considered legal documents and can be subject to audit; therefore, their integrity and accuracy must be ensured at all times. Any misuse of financial records associated with the practice can be considered fraud and abuse.

Student Name: _____ Date: _____

Time: Satisfactory   Unsatisfactory

Successful Completion: Yes   No

Grade/Points: _____   Pass   Fail

Need to Repeat: _____   Number of Attempts: 1   2   3

Instructor Comments: _____

_____

_____

CONDITIONS UNDER WHICH THE STUDENT IS EXPECTED TO PERFORM THE TASK

Follow Task/Performance Steps

Task/Performance Step	S	U
1. Student assembles equipment and supplies.		
2. Student totals cash and checks below. You have $1,040.00 in cash with NO coins. There is a bank charge of $10.00.		
3. Student lists all cash and checks separately on back of deposit slip and totals amount for each.		
4. Student writes in total amount of deposit on back of the deposit slip on the appropriate line.		
5. Student dates deposit slip.		
6. Student puts cash total for deposit on front of deposit slip on appropriate line.		
7. Student lists checks separately on the back of the deposit slip on the appropriate lines.		
8. Student totals amount of cash and checks on the front of the deposit slip on appropriate line.		
9. Student confirms totals on front and back of the deposit slip are equal.		
10. Student endorses checks provided with all required information. *"For Deposit Only" with physician's signature and account number ensures deposit into correct account and prevents unauthorized use of the check.*		
11. Student role-plays (pretends) to make copy of deposit slip.		
12. Student role-plays placing cash, endorsed checks, and deposit slip in deposit envelope.		
13. Student role-plays stapling deposit receipt to a copy of deposit slip and places in appropriate accounting journal.		
BANK RECONCILIATION		
14. Your bank statement came today. Student gathers necessary documentation and prepares the statement for reconciliation. • Prepare and maintain the bank statement by placing a check next to the items that have cleared. (Check numbers: 4560, 1191, 568, 4588) • Reconcile the statement using the attached reconciliation worksheet. Today's checks and cash are the only items not appearing on your statement. • Student writes in amount collected today that is not showing on statement: $1,040 cash, $100.00 check, $120.00 check on the enclosed bank reconciliation sheet.		
15. Student totals the deposits and documents on the appropriate line of the bank reconciliation sheet.		

16.	Student adds the total deposits to the balance per the bank statement and records on appropriate line.		
17.	Student adjusts bank balance by subtracting the outstanding check from the total balance.		
18.	Student writes in the bank charges and subtracts from the balance per checkbook.		
19.	Student records adjusted checkbook balance on appropriate line.		
20.	Student confirms that corrected checkbook balance is equal to the balance that shows in the bank statement (first line).		
21.	Student finds and corrects errors if the checkbook balance and the bank statement balance are not equal.		
22.	Student initials and dates bank reconciliation form on completion.		

Key: Satisfactory = S; Unsatisfactory = U

DEPOSIT SLIP FOR ACCOUNT OF

Dr. Franklin Pierce Wright
2310 Wright Way
Melbourne, FL 32904

Date _____ 20_____

Currency	
Cash	
Coin	
Total from other side	
NET DEPOSIT	

Community Bank
23 Group Drive
QC; FL 90167

     1 5 0 0 0 0 4: 0 0 8 5 :"

(Back of Deposit Slip)

Checks
List all items separately

Description (# or Name) | **Totals**

Totals
(Enter on Front Side)

BANK STATEMENT

Dr. Franklin Pierce Wright, Family Practice
2310 Wright Way
Melbourne, FL 32904

Checks

4560	$45.00	_____
1191	$15.00	_____
568	$25.00	_____
127	$100.00	_____
4588	$90.00	_____

The following 2 checks are for today's deposit. Don't forget to add in your cash. The third check is "outstanding" because it has not cleared on your bank statement.

Denny Stine   **6144**
31 Shore Drive
QC, Florida 90866   Date
                                          12/00/2005

Pay to the
Order of **Dr. Franklin Pierce Wright** $_____
One hundred and twenty and **xx** / **00** Dollars

PALM Bank
For **Office visit**   **Denny Stine**
:671284599   7713490976   6144

ENDORSE HERE

Do Not Sign/Write/Stamp Below This Line
For Financial Institution Use Only

Mary Manygrats
7 Poplar Drive
QC, Florida 90866

1368

Date
12/00/00

Pay to the
Order of **Dr. Franklin Pierce Wright** $100.00

One hundred and no/00 Dollars

PALM Bank

For _____

Mary Manygrats

:611234589 17813450976 1368

ENDORSE HERE

Do Not Sign/Write/Stamp Below This Line
For Financial Institution Use Only

OUTSTANDING CHECK

Shelby Minton
3110 Coral Reef Way
Palm Coast, FL 90169

127

Date 12/00/00

Pay to the
Order of **Dr. Franklin Wright Pierce** $ 100.00

One hundred and no cents Dollars

PALM Bank

For _____

Shelby Minton

671544511 4118950976 127

BANK RECONCILIATION WORKSHEET

December 23, 20xx

This is an example of the reverse side of the bank statement, which assists you in reconciling a checking account.

Enter:

The Bank Statement BALANCE that shows on the statement	$ 4,260.50
Minus the Outstanding Checks	$
Plus any Deposits not shown	$
Corrected Bank Statement Balance:	$
Checkbook Balance	$ 4,270.50
Less any Bank Charges	$
Correct Checkbook Balance	$

Initials:_____Date:_____

Practicum 16. Accounting Procedures

COMPETENCY

CAAHEP: 3. a. (2) (b) Post entries on a day sheet
3. a. (2) (c) Perform accounts receivable procedures
3. a. (2) (e) Post adjustments
3. a. (2) (f) Process credit balance
3. a. (2) (g) Process refunds
3. a. (2) (h) Post NSF checks
3. a. (2) (i) Post collection agency payments

ABHES: 3. (l) Post entries on a day sheet
3. (n) Prepare a check
3. (p) Post adjustments
3. (q) Process credit balance
3. (r) Process refunds
3. (s) Post NSF funds
3. (t) Post collection agency payments
8. (a) Use manual and computerized bookkeeping systems
8. (d) Manage accounts payable and receivable

SPECIFIC TASK

- Post 1 day's charges and payments (listed below) on the day sheet attached and post the same charges and payments on your medical office software. Follow the instructions provided from your computer software or instructions from your teacher.
- Post a batch insurance check received from the attached Prudential EOB (Explanation of Benefits) statement to the day sheet/computer provided. ROA (Received on Account).
- Process a credit balance for a patient with a refund, which is an adjustment to the account.
- Post an NSF check to the day sheet and computer.
- Post a collection agency check to the day sheet and computer.
- Complete the daily bookkeeping cycle, including total charges, total deposit, and proof of posting.

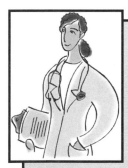

Make a Difference

Working with figures can be frustrating. You will have better success if you write neatly in the day sheet. Always double-check yourself the first time you enter numbers whether it is in the computer or manually. Most offices want the day sheet (total of the day's transactions) balanced before the employees can go home because the deposits are usually done on a daily basis. As the author, I can tell you that there were many times in my career that I had to stay late because the day sheet did not balance. It did not take long to realize that it is better to do it right the first time. Double-check your work!

STANDARD PRECAUTIONS

NA

EQUIPMENT/SUPPLIES

Pegboard/Day Sheet
Medical Office Accounting Software
Pen/Calculator
Attached list of cash and checks (ROAs)
Attached EOB
Attached Ledger Cards
Attached Blank Check

STANDARD OF PERFORMANCE OF THE TASK

You may earn a maximum of 5 points for each competency regardless of the number of steps to be performed.

    EX: If you miss two steps and achieve all the rest then you have earned 3 points.

    More than five steps missed means that you have 0 points.

    Your instructor may choose not to assign points but check you off on a pass or fail status.

Regardless, you may need to repeat the competency for successful completion.

    It is up to your instructor to determine the maximum number of tries before the competency has been met successfully in the time allotted.

Student Name: _____ Date: _____

Time: Satisfactory   Unsatisfactory

Successful Completion: Yes   No

Grade/Points: _____   Pass   Fail

Need to Repeat: _____ Number of Attempts: 1   2   3

Instructor Comments: _____

_____

_____

CONDITIONS UNDER WHICH THE STUDENT IS EXPECTED TO PERFORM THE TASK

Follow Task/Performance Steps

Task/Performance Step	S	U
ENTERING TRANSACTIONS ON DAY SHEET		
1. Student gathers needed financial documents and daily transactions. Turns on computer and sets up for entering data.		
2. Student obtains day sheet.		
3. Student reviews the day's transactions and remembers that all transactions added to the day sheet would also be added to the patient ledger both manually and in the computer.		
4. Student begins with patient Antonio Cann and proceeds with all patient entries, including charges, payments, and adjustments. Student records any previous and current balances. Student completes each row with the necessary information.		
5. Student forwards any previous days' balances in the designated space on day sheet.		
6. Student enters service code or description and fee in designated space on receipt.		
7. Student accepts and records patient's payment and new balance and records in appropriate columns.		
ENTERING CHECKS FROM PRUDENTIAL FROM THE EXPLANATION OF BENEFITS		
8. Student enters all check payments listed on EOB from insurance carrier. Student remembers to check previous balances from the two patients listed.		
9. Student enters the write-off adjustment for the designated patients listed under the adjustment column from the EOB. *Professional discounts and "write-offs" are commonly authorized by the physician as a courtesy to their patients for many reasons. When the physician is a provider, he/she must write off the difference between the charges and the allowed amount.*		
PROCESS THE REFUND CHECK		
10. When posting the Prudential payments student notices that patient Denny Stine has now overpaid. Student adds the refund to the day sheet as an adjustment and processes the refund check.		

NSF CHECK		
11. Student enters the NSF check following directions provided. *Patient accounts with a returned check for NSF usually will require also adding a check charge because the bank will most likely charge your account for the transaction. These types of transactions are posted as an adjustment while the check charge is posted as a charge. In the computer, your debit can serve as a credit and vice versa.*		
POSTING THE COLLECTION AGENCY CHECK		
12. Student posts the collection agency check to the day sheet. *Delinquent patient accounts collected by a collection agency must be documented on account as a payment reflected on the day sheet and patient ledger card.*		
13. Student totals all columns on the day sheet, using a pencil, in a timely manner and with accuracy.		
14. Student completes proof of totals and enters in ink on the day sheet. *Totaling proof columns ensures errors have not been made in calculation and your daily and monthly transactions are balanced.*		
15. Student continues the process until the day sheet is balanced.		

Key: Satisfactory = S; Unsatisfactory = U

Post on Day Sheet: This is a list of today's transactions. Date: 10/23/year

Name	Service	Charge	Payment	Adj.	PB	NB
Cann, Antonio	OV, MMR	65.00	65.00 ck (#4321)	0	45.00	45.00
Manygrats, Mary	OV ,UA	65.00	60.00 ck (#7641)	5.00	0	0
Plan, Marcus	OV, CBC	65.00	0	0	45.00	110.00
Quint, Patty	OV, Flu inj	60.00	30.00 csh	0	25.00	55.00
Kaine, Neil	OV, EKG	295.00	50.00 ck (#5164)	10.00	355.00	590.00
Swain, Ernest	OV, CXR	95.00	10.00 csh	0	20.00	105.00
Stine, Denny	OV, TC	50.00	75.00 ck (#6137)	0	95.00	70.00
Jonas, Quint	OV, Splint	75.00	20.00 csh	10.00	0	45.00
Minton, Shelby	OV, FBS	65.00	30.00 ck (#2165)	0	20.00	55.00
Burke, Ethel	OV, Hep B	60.00	0	0	40.00	100.00
Droflit, Phyllis	OV, CBC	65.00	20.00 csh	5.00	0	40.00
Droflit, Larry	MMR	25.00	25.00 ck (#3125)	0	0	0

| Rooso, Darcee | OV, Hct | 50.00 | 50.00
ck
(#2567) | 0 | 0 | 0 |

Key: Previous Balance = PB; New Balance = NB

ACCOUNTS WITH PREVIOUS BALANCES BEFORE EOB STATEMENT FROM PRUDENTIAL

These are mock ledger cards with previous balances to show you where you would find previous balances on patients. Be sure to add these balances to your day sheet before the insurance check below. Double check for other patient balances using the patient name and checking the day sheet for current balances.

Name:	Mary Manygrats	**DOB:**	02-20-45
Address:	980 Fern St.	**SS#:**	983-01-6385
	Palmetto, FL 90257	**Tel (H):**	512-777-2648
Insurance:	Prudential	**Emp:**	Carol's Hair Salon
	ID#: 2096482105	**Tel(W):**	512-779-2323
	Group#: 86206	**Spouse:**	Jim 06-11-44
		SS#:	267-81-5834

Patient's Name: Mary Manygrats

Statement to:

Date	Reference	Description	Charge	Credit Payment/Adjustment	Current Balance
				Balance Forward	65.00

Please Pay Amount in Last Column

Name: Neil Kaine   **DOB:** 12-23-47
Address: 710 Dolphin St.   **SS#:** 672-94-6382
Palmetto, FL 90257   **Tel (H):** 517-562-8365
Insurance: Prudential   **Emp:** Kaine Dry Cleaning
ID#: 9163064539   **Tel(W):** 517-568-9000
Group#: 73541   **Spouse:** Yoko 01-15-47
     SS#: 845-29-8210

Patient's Name: Neil Kane

Statement to:

Date	Reference	Description	Charge	Credit Payment/Adjustment	Current Balance
				Balance Forward	590.00

Please Pay Amount in Last Column

Batch check from Prudential. This amount must match the "Provider Paid" column below

Prudential   **4500**
1800 Insurance St.
Jacksonville, FL 91035   Date January 15, 20xx

Pay to the
Order of _____ Dr. Franklin Pierce Wright _____ $ _____ 270.00 _____

_____ Two Hundred and Seventy _____ Dollars

Forsythe Bank

For _____ Insurance Reimbursement _____   Jack Prudential

:497210864 820871460 4500

Prudential

PROVIDER STATEMENT OF EXPLANATION OF BENEFITS

Batch #042800

Patient Name	DOS	Charges	Allowed Amt.	Provider Paid	Adj.	Total
Antonio Cann	10-12	45.00	45.00	45.00	0	45.00
Denny Stine	10-23	95.00	55.00	55.00	40.00	55.00
Mary Manygrats	10-31	65.00	50.00	50.00	15.00	50.00
Neil Kaine	11-5	90.00	75.00	75.00	15.00	75.00
Marcus Plan	11-14	45.00	45.00	45.00	0	45.00

REFUND CHECK: ACCOUNTS PAYABLE

Denny Stine paid $75.00 in cash on 10-23. With the Prudential payment of $55 and the provider adjustment W/O of $40, Mr. Stine has overpaid by $25. Process refund check of $25.00. Add the refund to the day sheet as an adjustment. *Reminder*: **Mr. Stine already has a current balance of $70 that will now be the previous balance with this new entry.**

Dr. Franklin Pierce Wright , Family Practice	3451
2310 Wright Way	
Melbourne, FL 32904	Date _____

Pay to the
Order of _____ $ _____

_____ Dollars

Community Bank

For _____   _____

:298753098: 8624167849 3451

NSF CHECK

The following check received from Shelby Minton was returned due to NSF. Post to the day sheet as an adjustment. Post the $25.00 check charge from the bank in the charge column. Shelby Minton will have a current balance of $55.00. When posting, this amount becomes the patient's previous balance.

Shelby Minton	**2165**
3110 Coral Reef Way	
Palm Coast, FL 90169 **RETURNED FOR NSF**	Date 10/23/20xx

Pay to the
Order of __Dr. Franklin Pierce Wright__   **$ 30.00**

__Thirty_____and no cents_____ Dollars

PALM Bank

For _____   Shelby Minton

671544511 4118950976 127

CHECK RECEIVED FROM COLLECTION AGENCY

Post the following collection agency check to the day sheet. This patient has a previous balance of $500.00. The collection agency check is posted to the payment column. After posting you should see a new balance of $205.00

Collect Collection Agency	**5630**
54 Nuber Drive	
Tampa, FL 98452	Date January 10, 20xx

Pay to the
Order of _____Dr. Franklin Pierce Wright_____ $ _____

_____Two Hundred and Ninety-Five_____   00/100   Dollars

Harbor Bank

For __Neil Kaine_____

:753156290 8614309765 5630

Use the space provided to assist you with calculations or notes:

DAY SHEET DAILY BUSINESS SUMMARY

Daily log.

DAY SHEET DAILY BUSINESS SUMMARY

DAY SHEET (Daily Business Summary)

SHEET NO. _____ OF _____ DATE: _____

DATE	DESCRIPTION	CHARGE	CREDITS		CURRENT BALANCE	PREVIOUS BALANCE	NAME	RECEIPT NUMBER	CASH	CHECKS	BUSINESS ANALYSIS SUMMARIES (OPTIONAL)
			PAYMENTS	ADJ.							

Col. A   Col. B-1   Col. B-2   Col. C   Col.D

TOTALS THIS PAGE
PREVIOUS PAGE
MONTH-TO-DATE

TOTALS
CASH
CHECKS

PROOF OF POSTING

COL. D TOTAL	$
PLUS COL. A TOTAL	$
SUB TOTAL	$
LESS COLS. B-1 & B-2	$
MUST EQUAL COL.C	$

ACCOUNTS RECEIVABLE CONTROL

PREVIOUS DAY'S TOTAL	$
PLUS COL. A	$
SUB TOTAL	$
LESS COLS. B-1 & B-2	$
TOTAL ACCTS. REC.	$

ACCOUNTS RECEIVABLE PROOF

ACCTS. REC. 1ST OF MONTH	$
PLUS COL. A - MO. TO DATE	$
SUB TOTAL	$
LESS B-1 & B-2-MO. TO DATE	$
TOTAL ACCTS. REC.	$

CASH PAID OUT

	$
	$

CASH CONTROL

Beginning Cash On Hand	$
Receipts Today (Col. "B-1")	$
Total	$
Less Paid Outs	$
Less Bank Deposit	$
Closing Cash On Hand	$

Daily log.

Practicum 17. Billing and Collection

COMPETENCY

CAAHEP: 3. a. (2) (d) Perform billing and collection procedures
ABHES: 1. (h) Be courteous and diplomatic
2. (d) Serve as a liaison between the physician and others
3. (m) Perform billing and collection procedures
6. (f) Exercise efficient time management

SPECIFIC TASK

Exercising efficient time management skills as you process monthly billing statements and evaluate patient accounts for collection using the facility's collection policy (refer to Database).

Use courteous and diplomatic technique as you serve as a liaison between the patient and the physician.

Initiate proceedings for collection of delinquent accounts. Refer to attached Aging of Accounts Report.

STANDARD PRECAUTIONS

NA

EQUIPMENT/SUPPLIES

Database /report of past due patient accounts – attached
Statements (patient ledger cards) – attached
Computer/pen/telephone/medical assistant textbook

STANDARD OF PERFORMANCE OF THE TASK

You may earn a maximum of 5 points for each competency regardless of the number of steps to be performed.

EX: If you miss two steps and achieve all the rest then you have earned 3 points.

More than five steps missed means that you have 0 points.

Your instructor may choose not to assign points but check you off on a pass or fail status.
Regardless, you may need to repeat the competency for successful completion.

It is up to your instructor to determine the maximum number of tries before the competency has been met successfully in the time allotted.

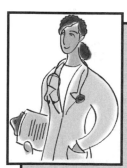

Make a Difference

Policy and procedure guidelines must be adhered to regarding debt collection. You are accountable for your actions as you serve as the physician's liaison. Refer to your textbook for guidelines when calling or sending collection notices and/or an example of a collection letter.

Student Name: _____   Date: _____

Time:	Satisfactory	Unsatisfactory
Successful Completion:	Yes	No
Grade/Points: _____	Pass	Fail
Need to Repeat: _____	Number of Attempts: 1 2 3	

Instructor Comments: _____

_____

_____

CONDITIONS UNDER WHICH THE STUDENT IS EXPECTED TO PERFORM THE TASK

Follow Task/Performance Steps

Task/Performance Step	S	U
1. Student assembles equipment and supplies.		
2. Student gathers and reviews all accounts with outstanding balances.		
3. Student prepares routine statements on a patient ledger card, including: • Date of preparation • Name and address of responsible party • Name of patient if different from responsible party • Itemized services • Unpaid balance		
4. Student separates delinquent accounts according to age account.		
5. Student determines and states action to be taken on each delinquent account using courteous and diplomatic writing skills.		
6. Student prepares cycle billing for appropriate accounts.		
7. Student documents cycle billing on patient ledger card.		
8. Student role-plays with a classmate and places necessary collection phone calls to accounts 90 days past due using courtesy and diplomacy.		
9. Student documents phone call and patients' responses on patient ledger card.		
10. Student prepares individual collection letter. Attach to appropriate page.		
11. Student documents on patient ledger that collection letter sent.		
12. Student demonstrated use of efficient time management skills by completing this task in the time specified by the instructor.		

Key: Satisfactory = S; Unsatisfactory = U

Aging of Accounts Report: December 30, 20xx

PATIENT NAME	ACCOUNT NUMBER	DUE DATE	AMOUNT
Accounts 30 Days Past Due:			
Ethel Burke	629-98-6301	12/10/00	45.00
Denny Stine	420-78-6310	12/14/00	75.00
Antonio Cann	438-00-7810	12/20/00	150.00
Accounts 60 Days Past Due:			
Mary Manygrats	983-01-6385	11/10/00	195.00
Patty Quint	483-81-5830	11/22/00	90.00
Accounts 90 Days Past Due:			
Marcus Plan	297-73-2784	10/15/00	50.00
Neil Kane	672-94-6382	10/25/00	45.00
Accounts 120 Days or More Past Due:			
Dan Had	519-52-7164	9/11/00	45.00
Total Overdue Accounts Receivable			**$695.00**

LEDGER CARDS

Name: Ethel Burke   **DOB:** 04-25-25
Address: 546 Dustin Ave.   **SS#:** 629-98-6301
Surfside, FL 90867   **Tel (H):** 568-321-7356
Insurance: Medicare   **Emp:** Retired
ID#: 629986301C   **Tel(W):** NA
Group#: 61842   **Spouse:** Samuel 11-21-24
    SS#: 510-52-7350

Patient's Name: Ethel Burke

Statement to:

Date	Reference	Description	Charge	Credit Payment/Adjustment	Current Balance
				Balance Forward	
12/10/00		OV Focuse	45.00	——————	45.00

Please Pay Amount in Last Column

Name: Denny Stine   **DOB:** 08-10-77

Address: 3434 Burch St.   **SS#:** 420-78-6310

Palmetto, FL 90256   **Tel (H):** 561-567-5061

Insurance: Blue Cross/ Blue Shield   **Emp:** Cosmos Hair

ID#: 1290765430   **Tel(W):** 561-568-0090

Group#: 495201   **Spouse:** NA

Patient's Name: Denny Stine

Statement to:

Date	Reference	Description	Charge	Credit Payment/Adjustment	Current Balance
				Balance Forward	
12/14/00		OV Expand	75.00		75.00

Please Pay Amount in Last Column

Name: Antonio Cann   **DOB:** 10-20-27
Address: 2300 Ocean Way   **SS#:** 438-00-7810
    Surfside, FL 90866   **Tel (H):** 561-778-7329
Insurance: Medicare   **Emp:** Retired
    ID#: 438007810C   **Tel(W):** NA
    Group#: 45001   **Spouse:** Franchesca 11-14-30
    SS#: 719-41-7830

Patient's Name: Antonio Cann

Statement to:

Date	Reference	Description	Charge	Credit Payment/Adjustment	Current Balance
				Balance Forward	
12/20/00		OV Comp, EKG 12-	150.00	————	150.00

Please Pay Amount in Last Column

Name: Mary Manygrats   **DOB:** 02-20-45

Address: 980 Fern St.   **SS#:** 983-01-6385

Palmetto, FL 90257   **Tel (H):** 512-777-2648

Insurance: Prudential   **Emp:** Carol's Hair Salon

ID#: 2096482105   **Tel(W):** 512-779-2323

Group#: 86206   **Spouse:** Jim 06-11-44

SS#: 267-81-5834

Patient's Name: Mary Manygrats

Statement to:

Date	Reference	Description	Charge	Credit Payment/Adjustment	Current Balance
				Balance Forward	100.00
11/10/00		OV Comprehensive	95.00	——	195.00

Please Pay Amount in Last Column

Name: Patty Quint   **DOB:** 03-28-71
Address: 60 Hibiscus Ct.   **SS#:** 483-81-5830
Surfside, FL 90866   **Tel (H):** 561-568-3810
Insurance: Blue Cross/Blue Shield   **Emp:** Bonns Realestate
ID#: 3901743829   **Tel(W):** 907-561-8181
Group#: 49015   **Spouse:** William 09-08-70
SS#: 109-45-8267

Patient's Name: Patty Quint

Statement to:

Date	Reference	Description	Charge	Credit Payment/Adjustment	Current Balance
				Balance Forward	
11/22/00		OV Expand	90.00	————	90.00

Please Pay Amount in Last Column

Name: Marcus Plan   **DOB:** 10-08-29
Address: 450 Windemere Pl.   **SS#:** 297-73-2784
Palm Coast, FL 90169   **Tel (H):** 907-286-5672
Insurance: Medicare   **Emp:** Retired
ID#: 297732784A   **Tel(W):** NA
Group#: 72195   **Spouse:** Audra 09-22-31
SS#: 490-38-1298

Patient's Name: Marcus Plan

Statement to:

Date	Reference	Description	Charge	Credit Payment/Adjustment	Current Balance
				Balance Forward	
10/15/00		OV, Glucos	50.00	————	50.00

Please Pay Amount in Last Column

Name: Neil Kaine   **DOB:** 12-23-47
Address: 710 Dolphin St.   **SS#:** 672-94-6382
    Palmetto, FL 90257   **Tel (H):** 517-562-8365
Insurance: Prudential   **Emp:** Kaine Dry Cleaning
    ID#: 9163064539   **Tel(W):** 517-568-9000
    Group#: 73541   **Spouse:** Yoko 01-15-47
    SS#: 845-29-8210

Patient's Name: Neil Kane

Statement to:

Date	Reference	Description	Charge	Credit Payment/Adjustment	Current Balance
				Balance Forward	
10/25/00		OV Focuse	45.00	——	45.00

Please Pay Amount in Last Column

Name: Dan Had   **DOB:** 05-21-73

Address: 571 East St.   **SS#:** 519-52-7164

Palm Coast, FL 90168   **Tel (H):** 907 561-6523

Insurance: Aetna   **Emp:** Harr Electronics

ID#: NA   **Tel(W):** 906-568-6190

Group#: 61893   **Spouse:** Karan 09-17-73

SS#: 459-61-5398

Dependents: Justin DOB: 11-13-96

Joanne DOB: 08-24-97

Jennifer DOB: 01-25-98

Jake DOB: 05-04-00

Patient's Name: Dan Had

Statement to:

Date	Reference	Description	Charge	Credit Payment/Adjustment	Current Balance
				Balance Forward	
9/11/00		OV Comprehensive	95.00	50.00/ 0.00	45.00

Please Pay Amount in Last Column

Attach collection letter to this page.

Practicum 18. Third-Party Management

COMPETENCY

CAAHEP: 3. a. (3) (b) Apply third-party guidelines

              3. c. (1) (a) Respond to and initiate written communication

ABHES: 2. (h) Receive, organize, prioritize, and transmit information expediently

              2. (o) Fundamental writing skills

              8. (c) Analyze and use current third-party guidelines for reimbursement

SPECIFIC TASK

Analyze and apply third-party guidelines by organizing the information and prioritizing and transmitting the response by written communication to the party requesting the information using the following scenario.

You have received correspondence requesting information about a patient from a third-party caller/insurance who is BC/BS.

The patient was involved in an automobile accident. The patient has two medical insurance companies. State Fame is the primary payer in this case and State Fame Auto Insurance becomes the third.

In the time specified by your instructor follow the task steps. How will you apply third-party guidelines and what will you do?

STANDARD PRECAUTIONS

NA

EQUIPMENT/SUPPLIES

Correspondence from BC/BS

Patient insurance card for verification

Written letter of response

Pen (paper attached)

STANDARD OF PERFORMANCE OF THE TASK

You may earn a maximum of 5 points for each competency regardless of the number of steps to be performed.

EX: If you miss two steps and achieve all the rest then you have earned 3 points.

More than five steps missed means that you have 0 points.

Your instructor may choose not to assign points but check you off on a pass or fail status.

Regardless, you may need to repeat the competency for successful completion.

It is up to your instructor to determine the maximum number of tries before the competency has been met successfully in the time allotted.

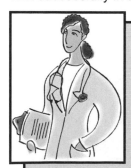

Make a Difference

Third-party Guideline

The patient must authorize requests from third-party callers or payers that are requesting financial or medical record information. This must be done by written permission from the patient.

Student Name: _____   Date: _____

Time: Satisfactory   Unsatisfactory

Successful Completion: Yes   No

Grade/Points: _____   Pass   Fail

Need to Repeat: _____   Number of Attempts: 1   2   3

Instructor Comments: _____

_____

_____

CONDITIONS UNDER WHICH THE STUDENT IS EXPECTED TO PERFORM THE TASK

Follow Task/Performance Steps

	Task/Performance Step	S	U
1.	Student obtains and reads correspondence from BC/BS.		
2.	Student organizes and prioritizes the information by applying third-party guidelines. Student lists what can and/or cannot be done with requests.		
3.	Student confirms BC/BS is a third-party payer by role-playing a call to BC/BS from the card on file.		
4.	Student attempts (role-play) to reach the patient to transmit information and request a written release of information. The patient does not give permission.		
5.	On the blank page provided, the student writes a letter to the party requesting the information.		
6.	The student addressed third-party guidelines in the written correspondence.		
7.	Student writes the correspondence professionally and neatly.		

Key: Satisfactory = S; Unsatisfactory = U

CORRESPONDENCE

Blu Cros/Blu Shield
P.O. Box 5569
Loon, MN 23900-4500

January 23, Year

Dr. Franklin Pierce Wright
2310 Wright Way
Melbourne, FL 32904

Dear Dr. Wright,

We are trying to process a claim on behalf of your patient, Josephine Matoral. We have received several letters from attorneys also requesting the same information.

We have not been successful in reaching Ms. Matoral to obtain clarification on the following issues:

1. Correct DOB.

2. Does she have other insurance?

3. Has her automobile insurance paid a portion of the claim? (It is our understanding from the automobile insurance that a check was delivered to her home.) We are not able to gather this information and thought perhaps she had paid you with this check for a portion of services rendered.

4. Do you have her maiden name in your file?

5. Lastly, we are confused if Davie R. Night, PA – Attorney at Law is her lawyer or the defense lawyer and were hoping you would have letters verifying this information.

Your reply and any information you can provide will be most helpful. You may send your responses to the above address.

Thank you for your time.

Jonathon Candonowrong
Accounting Representative

BC/BS/jc

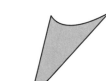

Prioritize and Organize Information

_____

_____

_____

_____

_____

_____

_____

_____

_____

_____

BCBS   Miami/Minnesota
Affiliates Network

Health Options Care Plan Inc.
Group # 73541
Electronic Payer ID 76240
672 94 6382 01
Josephine Matoral

% Payment only after verification all other coverage as paid.
South Florida Health Care Network – Loon, MN

PCP: Franklin Pierce Wright, MD - 1-800-565-3200

All covered nonemergency services must be billed through the subscriber's primary and secondary insurances before this insurance will cover any remainder. In case of illness or injury, contact your Primary Care Physician first. In case of medical emergency, which may be life threatening or cause serious bodily harm, get medical care immediately; then notify your primary care physician or call customer service within 48 hours. Refer to your member handbook for more information. Additional questions should be directed to customer service at the number listed on the front of this card. If you are traveling away from home and require medical care call the BCBS Health Care National Hotline at **1-800-381-5000**.
NOTICE TO ALL HEALTH CARE PROVIDERS:
This card is not a guarantee of coverage. For more information concerning coverage, copayment, and claim instruction, call customer service at the number listed on this side of card.

LETTER WRITTEN BY STUDENT

_____

_____

_____

_____

_____

_____

_____

_____

_____

_____

_____

_____

_____

_____

_____

_____

_____

_____

_____

_____

_____

_____

_____

_____

_____

_____

_____

Practicum 19. Insurance/Coding

COMPETENCY

CAAHEP: 3. a. (3) (c) Perform procedural coding
                 3. a. (3) (d) Perform diagnostic coding
                 3. a. (3) (e) Complete insurance claim forms
ABHES: 3. (w) Perform diagnostic coding
                 3. (x) Complete insurance claim forms
                 3. (y) Use physician fee schedule
                 8. (b) Implement current procedural terminology and ICD-9 coding

SPECIFIC TASK

Using the physician's fee schedule listed in the Database, implement and perform procedural and diagnostic coding by completing an insurance claim (CMS 1500) form. (Your instructor may vary the competency by having you perform these tasks on your medical office software in addition to the manual form [computer]).

STANDARD PRECAUTIONS

NA

EQUIPMENT/SUPPLIES

Black pen
Patient information form
Super bill (obtain from instructor)
Insurance form/CMS 1500 (obtain from instructor)

STANDARD OF PERFORMANCE OF THE TASK

You may earn a maximum of 5 points for each competency regardless of the number of steps to be performed.
    EX: If you miss two steps and achieve all the rest then you have earned 3 points.
    More than five steps missed means that you have 0 points.
    Your instructor may choose not to assign points but check you off on a pass or fail status.
Regardless, you may need to repeat the competency for successful completion.
    It is up to your instructor to determine the maximum number of tries before the competency has been met successfully in the time allotted.

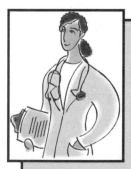

Make a Difference

Charges that you file on an insurance claim form would appear on the patient superbill and will show what services were performed and what the charges are for those services for the patient on a given day. There are many different types of terminology used to address a "superbill," such as "router," "fee-ticket," and "charge slip." Clinics/offices in different areas of the country will use a variety of terms but they all mean the same thing.

Student Name: _____   Date: _____

Time: Satisfactory   Unsatisfactory

Successful Completion: Yes   No

Grade/Points: _____   Pass   Fail

Need to Repeat: _____   Number of Attempts: 1   2   3

Instructor Comments: _____

_____

_____

CONDITIONS UNDER WHICH THE STUDENT IS EXPECTED TO PERFORM THE TASK

Follow Task/Performance Steps

Task/Performance Step	S	U
1. Student checks patient insurance in box 1 on the CMS 1500 insurance claim form.		
2. Student completes boxes 2–5 on the CMS form. Obtains the insured's ID number from the Patient Information Form.		
3. Student checks appropriate box for item 6.		
4. Student completes lines 7–11.		
5. Student completes lines 12 and 13 by writing "signature on file."		
6. Student writes N/A (not applicable) for items 14–19 unless case is related to an accident, injury, or pregnancy.		
7. Student completes items 20–22 as applicable.		
8. Student completes item 23 by correctly identifying the primary diagnosis code.		
9. Student completes item 24, A–G. For E: Identify diagnosis code by writing in the number in item 21 in which the code is listed.		
10. Student skips item 24H. The insurance company completes this line item.		
11. Student completes items 25–27 by referring to database.		
12. Student totals the charges and records on line 28.		
13. Student completes items 29–30. A co-payment of $15.00 has been collected.		
14. Student completes item 31 by having a classmate pose as the physician and requesting a signature. *Many offices use a stamp or the claims are electronically submitted.*		
15. Student identifies item 32 if applicable.		
16. Student reviews HCFA form for errors or omissions. *Never leave items blank. Enter "NA" if the item number does not pertain to the claim.*		
17. Student verifies insurance carrier address and places information in the upper right top of form.		

Key: Satisfactory = S; Unsatisfactory = U

Use the patient information listed below and on the patient information form to assist you in completing the insurance claim form and the encounter form. Complete the encounter form first.

Patient Account Number: ku456
Date of Service: January 24, Year
Diagnosis: Well-Adult Health Examination

Use the following services/charges with CPT and ICD-9 codes found in the Database or from codes assigned to you by your instructor from the coding books to complete the encounter form.

- Office Visit/NP – Complex
- EKG 12 Lead
- Spirometry Test
- CBC
- Influenza Injection

PATIENT INFORMATION
Please Print Clearly

Name ___Neil Kaine___   SS# _____672-94-6382_____
Address _710 Dolphin St.____   DL# ____K200798134____
City ____Palmetto____   State FL___ Zip 90257_____
Phone ___(517)562-8365_____   Birthdate __12/23/57_ Age _47_ Gender _M_
Married _X_____Single_____Divorced_____Widowed_____Separated_____
Employer __Kaine Dry Cleaning___ Occupation Self Employed___
Address_ 81 Surfside Blvd., Palmetto FL.__ Phone___(517)568-9000___
Insurance _Prudential____   ID#____9163064539____
Address _300 Marion Drive_____ Grp#_____73541_____
        _Longwood, FL._____ Phone _(800)348-2000___
Referred By:_____N/A_____

Responsible Party/Insured/Subscriber: _____Self_____

SPOUSE:
Name___Yokum_____   SS#_____845-29-8210_____
Address _same_____ DL#_____K20013889_____
City _____ State _____ Zip _____
Phone___same_____ Birthdate _1/15/57_ Age _47_ Gender _F_
Employer Self Employed_____ Occupation _____
Address_Same_____ Phone____same_____
Insurance Same as above_____ ID#_____9163064539-1___
Address _____ Grp#_____73541_____
        _____ Phone_____same_____

OTHER: Insured ____N/A_____ Relationship _____
Insurance_____ ID# _____
Address _____ Grp#_____
        _____ Phone_____

I understand that I am responsible for all charges not paid by my insurance company. I authorize the release of information for insurance billing and assign all benefits to
_____Dr. Franklin Pierce Wright_____.

_____**Neil Kaine**_____   ____January 24, 2005_____
Signature   Date

POST VISIT PLEASE RETURN THIS FORM TO THE RECEPTIONIST

Dr. Franklin Pierce Wright
Family Practice
2310 Wright Way
Melbourne, FL 32904
321 796-4440

State Lic # G46789
Fed ID # 59-8710766

☐Private   ☐BCBS   ☐Medicare   ☐Medicaid   ☐HMO   ☐Tricare   ☐Other   ☐Prudential

Patient's Last Name _____ First _____	Sex Today's Date ☐Male ☐Female _____/_____/_____
Address _____ _____ City _____ State _____ Zip _____	Relation to Subscriber Birthdate _____ _____/_____/_____
Subscriber or Guarantor	Insurance Carrier
Visit Related to Date of Onset ☐Illness ☐Pregnancy _____/_____/_____ ☐Work Injury ☐MVA	Insurance ID # Group
Subscriber Place of Employment (Address and Phone Number)	Other Health Coverage? ☐No ☐Yes (Identify below.)
Assignment: **I hereby assign my insurance benefits to be paid directly to the undersigned physician. I am financially responsible for non-covered services.** Signed: _____ Date _____ (Patient or Parent if Minor)	*Release:* **I authorize the undersigned physician to release any information acquired in the course of my examination or treatment.** Signed: _____ Date _____ (Patient or Parent if Minor)

CPT-Codes/Fee/Service

New Patient		Fee	Immunizations		Fee	Laboratory (in office)		Fee
Visit Level I	☐99201	_____	DTP	☐90701	_____	Pap Smear	☐88150	_____
Visit Level II	☐99202	_____	DT	☐90702	_____	Blood Sugar	☐82948	_____
Visit Level III	☐99203	_____	Tetanus	☐90703	_____	Hemoccult	☐82270	_____
Visit Level IV	☐99204	_____	OPV	☐90712	_____	UA, dipstick	☐81002	_____
Visit Level V	☐99205	_____	MMR	☐90707	_____	Urine Preg Test	☐81025	_____
Preventative Care			HIB	☐90647	_____	KOH slide	☐87220	_____
Infant (<1 yr)	☐99381	_____	Hep B	☐90746	_____	Rapid Strep	☐87880	_____
Child (1-4 yr)	☐99382	_____	Influenza	☐90658	_____	Wet Mount	☐87210	_____
Child (5-11 yr)	☐99383	_____	Pneumo	☐90732	_____	Hemoglobin	☐85018	_____
Child (12-17 yr)	☐99384	_____	TB Tine	☐86585	_____	CBC	☐85027	_____
18 – 39 years	☐99385	_____	**Injection Admin**			Venipuncture	☐36415	_____
40 – 64 years	☐99386	_____	Antibiotic, IM	☐90788	_____	Handling/Collection	☐99000	_____
65 + years	☐99387	_____	Therapeutic	☐90782	_____	Surgical Tray	☐99070	_____
Established Patient			Immun, single	☐90471	_____	Other	☐_____	_____
Visit Level I	☐99211	_____	Immun, ea addtl	☐90472	_____		☐_____	_____
Visit Level II	☐99212	_____	**Procedures**				☐_____	_____
Visit Level III	☐99213	_____	Anoscopy	☐46600	_____		☐_____	_____
Visit Level IV	☐99214	_____	Audiometry	☐92551	_____			
Visit Level V	☐99215	_____	Avul/Nail	☐11730	_____			
Diagnostic X-ray			Burn Tx	☐16020	_____			
Clavicle	☐73000	_____	I&D	☐10060	_____			
Shoulder/3 views	☐73030	_____	EKG	☐93000	_____			
Forearm	☐73090	_____	Ear Lavage	☐69210	_____			
Wrist	☐73110	_____	Spirometry	☐94010	_____			
Ankle	☐73610	_____						
Chest/2 views	☐71020	_____						

ICD-9-CM Codes

□ Abscess	682.9	□ Contraception	V25.09	□ Lymphadenopathy	289.3
□ Abrasion-Sup.Injury	919	□ Cough	786.2	□ Nausea/Vomiting	787.0
□ Acne	706.1	□ CVA	436.0	□ Obesity	278.0
□ Allergic Reaction	995.3	□ Depression	311	□ Osteoporosis	733.00
□ Amenorrhea	626.0	□ Dermatitis	692.9	□ Pharyngitis	462.0
□ Anemia	285.9	□ Diabetes*	250.00	□ Pneumonia	486.0
□ Anxiety	300.0	□ Dysmenorrhea	625.3	□ Pregnancy	V22.2
□ Annual GYN exam	V72.31	□ Ear Impaction	380.4	□ Rectal Bleed	569.3
□ Annual PE	V70.0	□ Fatigue	780.7	□ Sinusitis	461.9
□ Arrhythmia	427.9	□ Fever	780.6	□ STD _____	
□ Arthritis	716.9	□ Fracture	_____	□ Tendonitis	726.90
□ ASHD	414.0	□ Gastritis	535.0	□ UTI	599.0
□ Asthma	493.0	□ Gastroenteritis	558.9	□ URI	465.9
□ Backache	724.5	□ Gout	274.9	□ Vaginitis	616.1
□ Breast Mass	611.72	□ Headache	784.0	□ Well Baby/Child	V20.2
□ Bronchitis	490.0	□ Hematuria	599.7	□ Weight Loss	783.2
□ Bursitis	727.3	□ Hemorrhoids	455.6	□ Otitis Media	382.9
□ CAD	414.0	□ HIV	042	□ _____	_____
□ Chest Pain	786.5	□ Hypertension	401.9	□ _____	_____
□ CHF	428.0	□ Hypothyroidism	244.9	□ _____	_____
□ Conjunctivitis	372.3	□ IBS	787.5	□ _____	_____
□ COPD	496.0	□ Low Back Pain	724.2		

Return Appointment: _____

Physician Signature: _____

Previous Bal: _____

Total Charges: _____

Total: _____

Amt Recd: _____ □ cash □check (#____)
□credit card

New Balance: _____

CMS 1500 INSURANCE FORM

PLEASE
DO NOT
STAPLE
IN THIS
AREA

CARRIER

| PICA | | HEALTH INSURANCE CLAIM FORM | PICA | |

1. MEDICARE (Medicare #) **MEDICAID** (Medicaid #) **CHAMPUS** (Sponsor's SSN) **CHAMPVA** (VA File #) **GROUP HEALTH PLAN** (SSN or ID) **FECA BLK LUNG** (SSN) **OTHER** (ID)   **1a. INSURED'S I.D. NUMBER** (FOR PROGRAM IN ITEM 1)

2. PATIENT'S NAME (Last Name, First Name, Middle Initial)   **3. PATIENT'S BIRTH DATE** MM | DD | YY **SEX** M F   **4. INSURED'S NAME** (Last Name, First Name, Middle Initial)

5. PATIENT'S ADDRESS (No., Street)   **6. PATIENT RELATIONSHIP TO INSURED** Self Spouse Child Other   **7. INSURED'S ADDRESS** (No., Street)

CITY   **STATE**   **8. PATIENT STATUS** Single Married Other   Employed Full-Time Student Part-Time Student   **CITY**   **STATE**

ZIP CODE   **TELEPHONE** (Include Area Code) ( )   **ZIP CODE**   **TELEPHONE (INCLUDE AREA CODE)** ( )

9. OTHER INSURED'S NAME (Last Name, First Name, Middle Initial)   **10. IS PATIENT'S CONDITION RELATED TO:**   **11. INSURED'S POLICY GROUP OR FECA NUMBER**

a. OTHER INSURED'S POLICY OR GROUP NUMBER   **a. EMPLOYMENT? (CURRENT OR PREVIOUS)** YES NO   **a. INSURED'S DATE OF BIRTH** MM | DD | YY **SEX** M F

b. OTHER INSURED'S DATE OF BIRTH MM | DD | YY **SEX** M F   **b. AUTO ACCIDENT?** YES NO **PLACE (State)**   **b. EMPLOYER'S NAME OR SCHOOL NAME**

c. EMPLOYER'S NAME OR SCHOOL NAME   **c. OTHER ACCIDENT?** YES NO   **c. INSURANCE PLAN NAME OR PROGRAM NAME**

d. INSURANCE PLAN NAME OR PROGRAM NAME   **10d. RESERVED FOR LOCAL USE**   **d. IS THERE ANOTHER HEALTH BENEFIT PLAN?** YES NO *If yes,* return to and complete item 9 a-d.

READ BACK OF FORM BEFORE COMPLETING & SIGNING THIS FORM.
12. PATIENT'S OR AUTHORIZED PERSON'S SIGNATURE I authorize the release of any medical or other information necessary to process this claim. I also request payment of government benefits either to myself or to the party who accepts assignment below.
SIGNED _____ DATE _____

13. INSURED'S OR AUTHORIZED PERSON'S SIGNATURE I authorize payment of medical benefits to the undersigned physician or supplier for services described below.
SIGNED _____

PATIENT AND INSURED INFORMATION

14. DATE OF CURRENT: ILLNESS (First symptom) OR INJURY (Accident) OR PREGNANCY(LMP) MM | DD | YY   **15. IF PATIENT HAS HAD SAME OR SIMILAR ILLNESS.** GIVE FIRST DATE MM | DD | YY   **16. DATES PATIENT UNABLE TO WORK IN CURRENT OCCUPATION** MM | DD | YY FROM TO MM | DD | YY

17. NAME OF REFERRING PHYSICIAN OR OTHER SOURCE   **17a. I.D. NUMBER OF REFERRING PHYSICIAN**   **18. HOSPITALIZATION DATES RELATED TO CURRENT SERVICES** MM | DD | YY FROM TO MM | DD | YY

19. RESERVED FOR LOCAL USE   **20. OUTSIDE LAB?** YES NO **$ CHARGES**

21. DIAGNOSIS OR NATURE OF ILLNESS OR INJURY. (RELATE ITEMS 1,2,3 OR 4 TO ITEM 24E BY LINE)
1. |___ . ___   3. |___ . ___
2. |___ . ___   4. |___ . ___

22. MEDICAID RESUBMISSION CODE **ORIGINAL REF. NO.**

23. PRIOR AUTHORIZATION NUMBER

24. A DATE(S) OF SERVICE From MM DD YY To MM DD YY	B Place of Service	C Type of Service	D PROCEDURES, SERVICES, OR SUPPLIES (Explain Unusual Circumstances) CPT/HCPCS MODIFIER	E DIAGNOSIS CODE	F $ CHARGES	G DAYS OR UNITS	H EPSDT Family Plan	I EMG	J COB	K RESERVED FOR LOCAL USE
1										
2										
3										
4										
5										
6										

25. FEDERAL TAX I.D. NUMBER SSN EIN   **26. PATIENT'S ACCOUNT NO.**   **27. ACCEPT ASSIGNMENT?** (For govt. claims, see back) YES NO   **28. TOTAL CHARGE** $ **29. AMOUNT PAID** $ **30. BALANCE DUE** $

31. SIGNATURE OF PHYSICIAN OR SUPPLIER INCLUDING DEGREES OR CREDENTIALS (I certify that the statements on the reverse apply to this bill and are made a part thereof.)
SIGNED _____ DATE _____

32. NAME AND ADDRESS OF FACILITY WHERE SERVICES WERE RENDERED (If other than home or office)

33. PHYSICIAN'S, SUPPLIER'S BILLING NAME, ADDRESS, ZIP CODE & PHONE #
PIN# GRP#

PHYSICIAN OR SUPPLIER INFORMATION

(APPROVED BY AMA COUNCIL ON MEDICAL SERVICE 8/88) **PLEASE PRINT OR TYPE** APPROVED OMB-0938-0008 FORM CMS-1500 (12/90), FORM RRB-1500, APPROVED OMB-1215-0055 FORM OWCP-1500, APPROVED OMB-0720-0001 (CHAMPUS)

CMS-1500 sample provided by Provistas, Incorporated *http://www.medical-coding.net*

BECAUSE THIS FORM IS USED BY VARIOUS GOVERNMENT AND PRIVATE HEALTH PROGRAMS, SEE SEPARATE INSTRUCTIONS ISSUED BY APPLICABLE PROGRAMS.

NOTICE: Any person who knowingly files a statement of claim containing any misrepresentation or any false, incomplete or misleading information may be guilty of a criminal act punishable under law and may be subject to civil penalties.

REFERS TO GOVERNMENT PROGRAMS ONLY

MEDICARE AND CHAMPUS PAYMENTS: A patient's signature requests that payment be made and authorizes release of any information necessary to process the claim and certifies that the information provided in Blocks 1 through 12 is true, accurate and complete. In the case of a Medicare claim, the patient's signature authorizes any entity to release to Medicare medical and nonmedical information, including employment status, and whether the person has employer group health insurance, liability, no-fault, worker's compensation or other insurance which is responsible to pay for the services for which the Medicare claim is made. See 42 CFR 411.24(a). If item 9 is completed, the patient's signature authorizes release of the information to the health plan or agency shown. In Medicare assigned or CHAMPUS participation cases, the physician agrees to accept the charge determination of the Medicare carrier or CHAMPUS fiscal intermediary as the full charge, and the patient is responsible only for the deductible, coinsurance and noncovered services. Coinsurance and the deductible are based upon the charge determination of the Medicare carrier or CHAMPUS fiscal intermediary if this is less than the charge submitted. CHAMPUS is not a health insurance program but makes payment for health benefits provided through certain affiliations with the Uniformed Services. Information on the patient's sponsor should be provided in those items captioned in "Insured"; i.e., items 1a, 4, 6, 7, 9, and 11.

BLACK LUNG AND FECA CLAIMS

The provider agrees to accept the amount paid by the Government as payment in full. See Black Lung and FECA instructions regarding required procedure and diagnosis coding systems.

SIGNATURE OF PHYSICIAN OR SUPPLIER (MEDICARE, CHAMPUS, FECA AND BLACK LUNG)

I certify that the services shown on this form were medically indicated and necessary for the health of the patient and were personally furnished by me or were furnished incident to my professional service by my employee under my immediate personal supervision, except as otherwise expressly permitted by Medicare or CHAMPUS regulations.

For services to be considered as "incident" to a physician's professional service, 1) they must be rendered under the physician's immediate personal supervision by his/her employee, 2) they must be an integral, although incidental part of a covered physician's service, 3) they must be of kinds commonly furnished in physician's offices, and 4) the services of nonphysicians must be included on the physician's bills.

For CHAMPUS claims, I further certify that I (or any employee) who rendered services am not an active duty member of the Uniformed Services or a civilian employee of the United States Government or a contract employee of the United States Government, either civilian or military (refer to 5 USC 5536). For Black-Lung claims, I further certify that the services performed were for a Black Lung-related disorder.

No Part B Medicare benefits may be paid unless this form is received as required by existing law and regulations (42 CFR 424.32).

NOTICE: Any one who misrepresents or falsifies essential information to receive payment from Federal funds requested by this form may upon conviction be subject to fine and imprisonment under applicable Federal laws.

NOTICE TO PATIENT ABOUT THE COLLECTION AND USE OF MEDICARE, CHAMPUS, FECA, AND BLACK LUNG INFORMATION
(PRIVACY ACT STATEMENT)

We are authorized by CMS, CHAMPUS and OWCP to ask you for information needed in the administration of the Medicare, CHAMPUS, FECA, and Black Lung programs. Authority to collect information is in section 205(a), 1862, 1872 and 1874 of the Social Security Act as amended, 42 CFR 411.24(a) and 424.5(a) (6), and 44 USC 3101,41 CFR 101 et seq and 10 USC 1079 and 1086; 5 USC 8101 et seq; and 30 USC 901 et seq; 38 USC 613; E.O. 9397.

The information we obtain to complete claims under these programs is used to identify you and to determine your eligibility. It is also used to decide if the services and supplies you received are covered by these programs and to insure that proper payment is made.

The information may also be given to other providers of services, carriers, intermediaries, medical review boards, health plans, and other organizations or Federal agencies, for the effective administration of Federal provisions that require other third parties payers to pay primary to Federal program, and as otherwise necessary to administer these programs. For example, it may be necessary to disclose information about the benefits you have used to a hospital or doctor. Additional disclosures are made through routine uses for information contained in systems of records.

FOR MEDICARE CLAIMS: See the notice modifying system No. 09-70-0501, titled, 'Carrier Medicare Claims Record,' published in the Federal Register, Vol. 55 No. 177, page 37549, Wed. Sept. 12, 1990, or as updated and republished.

FOR OWCP CLAIMS: Department of Labor, Privacy Act of 1974, "Republication of Notice of Systems of Records," Federal Register Vol. 55 No. 40, Wed Feb. 28, 1990, See ESA-5, ESA-6, ESA-12, ESA-13, ESA-30, or as updated and republished.

FOR CHAMPUS CLAIMS: PRINCIPLE PURPOSE(S): To evaluate eligibility for medical care provided by civilian sources and to issue payment upon establishment of eligibility and determination that the services/supplies received are authorized by law.

ROUTINE USE(S): Information from claims and related documents may be given to the Dept. of Veterans Affairs, the Dept. of Health and Human Services and/or the Dept. of Transportation consistent with their statutory administrative responsibilities under CHAMPUS/CHAMPVA; to the Dept. of Justice for representation of the Secretary of Defense in civil actions; to the Internal Revenue Service, private collection agencies, and consumer reporting agencies in connection with recoupment claims; and to Congressional Offices in response to inquiries made at the request of the person to whom a record pertains. Appropriate disclosures may be made to other federal, state, local, foreign government agencies, private business entities, and individual providers of care, on matters relating to entitlement, claims adjudication, fraud, program abuse, utilization review, quality assurance, peer review, program integrity, third-party liability, coordination of benefits, and civil and criminal litigation related to the operation of CHAMPUS.

DISCLOSURES: Voluntary; however, failure to provide information will result in delay in payment or may result in denial of claim. With the one exception discussed below, there are no penalties under these programs for refusing to supply information. However, failure to furnish information regarding the medical services rendered or the amount charged would prevent payment of claims under these programs. Failure to furnish any other information, such as name or claim number, would delay payment of the claim. Failure to provide medical information under FECA could be deemed an obstruction.

It is mandatory that you tell us if you know that another party is responsible for paying for your treatment. Section 1128B of the Social Security Act and 31 USC 3801-3812 provide penalties for withholding this information.

You should be aware that P.L. 100-503, the "Computer Matching and Privacy Protection Act of 1988", permits the government to verify information by way of computer matches.

MEDICAID PAYMENTS (PROVIDER CERTIFICATION)

I hereby agree to keep such records as are necessary to disclose fully the extent of services provided to individuals under the State's Title XIX plan and to furnish information regarding any payments claimed for providing such services as the State Agency or Dept. of Health and Human Services may request.

I further agree to accept, as payment in full, the amount paid by the Medicaid program for those claims submitted for payment under that program, with the exception of authorized deductible, coinsurance, co-payment or similar cost-sharing charge.

SIGNATURE OF PHYSICIAN (OR SUPPLIER): I certify that the services listed above were medically indicated and necessary to the health of this patient and were personally furnished by me or my employee under my personal direction.

NOTICE: This is to certify that the foregoing information is true, accurate and complete. I understand that payment and satisfaction of this claim will be from Federal and State funds, and that any false claims, statements, or documents, or concealment of a material fact, may be prosecuted under applicable Federal or State laws.

According to the Paperwork Reduction Act of 1995, no persons are required to respond to a collection of information unless it displays a valid OMB control number. The valid OMB control number for this information collection is 0938-0008. The time required to complete this information collection is estimated to average 10 minutes per response, including the time to review instructions, search existing data resources, gather the data needed, and complete and review the information collection. If you have any comments concerning the accuracy of the time estimate(s) or suggestions for improving this form, please write to: CMS, Attn: PRA Reports Clearance Officer, 7500 Security Boulevard, Baltimore, Maryland 21244-1850.

CMS-1500 sample provided by Provistas, Incorporated *http://www.medical-coding.net*

CMS 1500 INSURANCE FORM

PLEASE
DO NOT
STAPLE
IN THIS
AREA

CARRIER →

| | PICA | | | | **HEALTH INSURANCE CLAIM FORM** | PICA | |

| 1. MEDICARE | MEDICAID | CHAMPUS | CHAMPVA | GROUP HEALTH PLAN | FECA BLK LUNG | OTHER | 1a. INSURED'S I.D. NUMBER (FOR PROGRAM IN ITEM 1) |
| (Medicare #) | (Medicaid #) | (Sponsor's SSN) | (VA File #) | (SSN or ID) | (SSN) | (ID) | |

2. PATIENT'S NAME (Last Name, First Name, Middle Initial)

3. PATIENT'S BIRTH DATE   MM   DD   YY   SEX   M   F

4. INSURED'S NAME (Last Name, First Name, Middle Initial)

5. PATIENT'S ADDRESS (No., Street)

6. PATIENT RELATIONSHIP TO INSURED   Self   Spouse   Child   Other

7. INSURED'S ADDRESS (No., Street)

CITY   STATE

8. PATIENT STATUS   Single   Married   Other   Employed   Full-Time Student   Part-Time Student

CITY   STATE

ZIP CODE   TELEPHONE (Include Area Code)   (   )

ZIP CODE   TELEPHONE (INCLUDE AREA CODE)   (   )

9. OTHER INSURED'S NAME (Last Name, First Name, Middle Initial)

10. IS PATIENT'S CONDITION RELATED TO:

11. INSURED'S POLICY GROUP OR FECA NUMBER

a. OTHER INSURED'S POLICY OR GROUP NUMBER

a. EMPLOYMENT? (CURRENT OR PREVIOUS)   YES   NO

a. INSURED'S DATE OF BIRTH   MM   DD   YY   SEX   M   F

b. OTHER INSURED'S DATE OF BIRTH   MM   DD   YY   SEX   M   F

b. AUTO ACCIDENT?   PLACE (State)   YES   NO

b. EMPLOYER'S NAME OR SCHOOL NAME

c. EMPLOYER'S NAME OR SCHOOL NAME

c. OTHER ACCIDENT?   YES   NO

c. INSURANCE PLAN NAME OR PROGRAM NAME

d. INSURANCE PLAN NAME OR PROGRAM NAME

10d. RESERVED FOR LOCAL USE

d. IS THERE ANOTHER HEALTH BENEFIT PLAN?   YES   NO   *If yes,* return to and complete item 9 a-d.

READ BACK OF FORM BEFORE COMPLETING & SIGNING THIS FORM.
12. PATIENT'S OR AUTHORIZED PERSON'S SIGNATURE I authorize the release of any medical or other information necessary to process this claim. I also request payment of government benefits either to myself or to the party who accepts assignment below.

SIGNED _____   DATE _____

13. INSURED'S OR AUTHORIZED PERSON'S SIGNATURE I authorize payment of medical benefits to the undersigned physician or supplier for services described below.

SIGNED _____

PATIENT AND INSURED INFORMATION

14. DATE OF CURRENT: ILLNESS (First symptom) OR INJURY (Accident) OR PREGNANCY(LMP)   MM   DD   YY

15. IF PATIENT HAS HAD SAME OR SIMILAR ILLNESS. GIVE FIRST DATE   MM   DD   YY

16. DATES PATIENT UNABLE TO WORK IN CURRENT OCCUPATION   FROM   MM   DD   YY   TO   MM   DD   YY

17. NAME OF REFERRING PHYSICIAN OR OTHER SOURCE

17a. I.D. NUMBER OF REFERRING PHYSICIAN

18. HOSPITALIZATION DATES RELATED TO CURRENT SERVICES   FROM   MM   DD   YY   TO   MM   DD   YY

19. RESERVED FOR LOCAL USE

20. OUTSIDE LAB?   YES   NO $ CHARGES

21. DIAGNOSIS OR NATURE OF ILLNESS OR INJURY. (RELATE ITEMS 1,2,3 OR 4 TO ITEM 24E BY LINE)

1. ____ . ____   3. ____ . ____

2. ____ . ____   4. ____ . ____

22. MEDICAID RESUBMISSION CODE   ORIGINAL REF. NO.

23. PRIOR AUTHORIZATION NUMBER

24. A						B	C	D	E	F	G	H	I	J	K
DATE(S) OF SERVICE						Place of Service	Type of Service	PROCEDURES, SERVICES, OR SUPPLIES (Explain Unusual Circumstances)	DIAGNOSIS CODE	$ CHARGES	DAYS OR UNITS	EPSDT Family Plan	EMG	COB	RESERVED FOR LOCAL USE
From			To					CPT/HCPCS MODIFIER							
MM	DD	YY	MM	DD	YY										
1															
2															
3															
4															
5															
6															

25. FEDERAL TAX I.D. NUMBER   SSN   EIN

26. PATIENT'S ACCOUNT NO.

27. ACCEPT ASSIGNMENT? (For govt. claims, see back)   YES   NO

28. TOTAL CHARGE $

29. AMOUNT PAID $

30. BALANCE DUE $

31. SIGNATURE OF PHYSICIAN OR SUPPLIER INCLUDING DEGREES OR CREDENTIALS (I certify that the statements on the reverse apply to this bill and are made a part thereof.)

SIGNED _____   DATE _____

32. NAME AND ADDRESS OF FACILITY WHERE SERVICES WERE RENDERED (If other than home or office)

33. PHYSICIAN'S, SUPPLIER'S BILLING NAME, ADDRESS, ZIP CODE & PHONE #

PIN#   GRP#

PHYSICIAN OR SUPPLIER INFORMATION

(APPROVED BY AMA COUNCIL ON MEDICAL SERVICE 8/88)   **PLEASE PRINT OR TYPE**   APPROVED OMB-0938-0008 FORM CMS-1500 (12/90),   FORM RRB-1500,   APPROVED OMB-1215-0055 FORM OWCP-1500,   APPROVED OMB-0720-0001 (CHAMPUS)

CMS-1500 sample provided by Provistas, Incorporated *http://www.medical-coding.net*

Practicum 20. Office Maintenance

COMPETENCY

CAAHEP: 3. c. (4) (a) Perform an inventory of supplies and equipment
3. c. (4) (b) Perform routine maintenance of administrative and clinical equipment
ABHES: 6. (a) Maintain physical plant
6. (b) Operate and maintain facilities and equipment safely
6. (c) Inventory equipment and supplies
6. (d) Evaluate and recommend equipment and supplies for practice
7. (d) Orient and train personnel

SPECIFIC TASK

Your instructor will assign you a section or stock area of the laboratory/classroom/storeroom. In the time specified by your instructor, complete an inventory of the assigned supplies and equipment. Once you have completed the inventory list, complete the recommended reorder form and recommend those supplies that need to be ordered.

Perform routine maintenance using the record form provided for you. Follow the steps below to ensure quality control on the equipment.

Once you have completed the above two tasks, role-play with a classmate and orient and train them to the importance of regular inventory of supplies and equipment and how to operate the equipment safely. Your instructor will assign one piece of equipment in which you will document how to use or operate this piece of equipment safely.

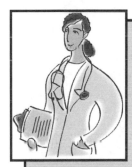

Make a Difference

To maintain the physical plant there are certain tasks that must be performed on a daily, monthly, and quarterly basis. Proper and frequent inventory of supplies and equipment is essential for the treatment and care of the patient. The use of manufacturer instructions is important to understand and ensure that routine maintenance is being conducted at regular intervals and that all equipment is in good working order. It is important to have on hand a Policy and Procedural Manual that will instruct an employee on how your office ensures maintenance of the physical plant. This will ensure safety for the physician, staff, and the patients. There is nothing more frustrating than needing a specific type of equipment or certain supplies during treatment or diagnostic testing, only to find that it has failed or the supplies you need are not there. Who suffers? The patient!

STANDARD PRECAUTIONS

Manufacturer safety instructions

EQUIPMENT/SUPPLIES

Various administrative/clinical equipment and supplies (Examples of Equipment: Autoclave, ECG Machine, and Computer)
Office policy/procedure manual if applicable (or instructions by your instructor)
Equipment Maintenance Record form
Equipment History form
Inventory form
Reorder form
Pen

STANDARD OF PERFORMANCE OF THE TASK

You may earn a maximum of 5 points for each competency regardless of the number of steps to be performed.

 EX: If you miss two steps and achieve all the rest then you have earned 3 points.

 More than five steps missed means that you have 0 points.

 Your instructor may choose not to assign points but check you off on a pass or fail status. Regardless, you may need to repeat the competency for successful completion.

 It is up to your instructor to determine the maximum number of tries before the competency has been met successfully in the time allotted.

Student Name: _____   Date: _____

Time: Satisfactory   Unsatisfactory

Successful Completion: Yes   No

Grade/Points: _____   Pass   Fail

Need to Repeat: _____   Number of Attempts: 1   2   3

Instructor Comments: _____

_____

_____

CONDITIONS UNDER WHICH THE STUDENT IS EXPECTED TO PERFORM THE TASK

Follow Task/Performance Steps

Task/Performance Step	S	U
1. Using the Inventory Checklist and Reorder form list attached, check supplies and equipment present and those items that need to be ordered and restocked. Be sure to always look in boxes that appear half empty or half full. Report the number of cases by boxes or packages if the case is not full. Report equipment by the name, including the serial number: • ECG Machine(s) • Autoclave • Wall Ophthalmoscope/Otoscope Unit • Computer		
2. Complete the Equipment History Form.		
3. Complete the Maintenance Record Form by performing the monthly maintenance as follows and document on the form: • Check all electrical cords to ensure there is no fraying or malfunction. • Check all electrical plugs to ensure they are safe and hooked correctly. • Check the monitor or screens for cracks, dust, or other obvious impairments or malfunctions. • Check any back-up batteries or packs to ensure they are in working order. • Check any keyboards for cracks or numbers and letters that are becoming hard to distinguish. • Check for dust that settles in the key pads. • Check light sources and rechargeable batteries. • Check leads and wires. • Perform autoclave cleaning if applicable.		
4. Role-play with a classmate and call the appropriate repair offices if applicable and schedule a time for the maintenance of equipment that needs repairing. Show the list of supplies that need reordering to your instructor.		
5. Role-play with a classmate and train and orient policy and procedure. Have new employee sign the "New Employee Orientation Documentation."		

Key: Satisfactory = S; Unsatisfactory = U

Inventory Checklist – Supplies and Equipment Reorder Form

SUPPLIES

Supply Item	Quantity (EA,BX,CS)	Reorder – Quantity

EA – Each = EA; Box = BX; Case = CS

EQUIPMENT

Equipment	Serial #	Model #	Quantity	Reorder Quantity

Equipment History Form

Equipment _____ Date Checked _____

Model No. _____ Serial No. _____

Date Purchased _____

Manufacturer _____

Telephone _____ Contact Person _____

Dealer/Warranty _____

_____

Equipment Working Properly _____

Equipment Needs Maintenance/Repairing _____

Equipment Problem _____

Technical Service Representative _____

Telephone _____

Service Record, Comments, Who was contacted, action taken

_____

_____

_____

_____

_____

_____

_____

Date _____

Equipment Maintenance Record Form

Date	Activity	Last Date Checked	Action Taken?

ORIENTATION/TRAINING LOG

New Employee

Name _____ Date _____

I, _____, have read the Policy and Procedural Manual (Database) and have received instruction on how to safely operate and maintain all equipment both clinically and administratively.

Furthermore, I understand that it is the responsibility of each employee to report supplies and equipment that need reordering or in case of malfunction that I report to the supervisor immediately.

I also understand that I will be assigned routine tasks on a daily, weekly, and quarterly basis that will ensure the safety of the patients, staff, and the physician and that I will perform these duties faithfully.

_____
Signature of Employee

(This document becomes a part of the employee record and is kept in the Human Resource Department or Physician/Office Manager's office).

Practicum 21. Payroll

COMPETENCY

CAAHEP: NA
ABHES: 8. (f) Process employee payroll

SPECIFIC TASK

In the time specified by your instructor, process a 1-week payroll for your employee using the information provided. Complete the Wage Statement, Individual Payroll Record, and the employee check. The taxes withheld have already been calculated for you from the Withholding Tax Table and employer insurance policies. This employee has worked a 40-hour workweek with no overtime. Follow each task step carefully.

Employee Name: Stacy Wantsmoney, RMA
Social Security: 123-45-6789
Status: Single
Exemptions: One, Self
Payroll Period: January 1, 20xx, to January 5, 20xx
Wage: $12.00 hourly – Salary – No time card

Taxes Withheld: Fed. Income Tax: $118.28
Social Security: $104.33
Medicare: $24.40
State Income Tax: $26.68
Disability Insurance: $15.14

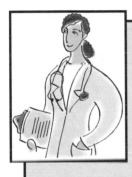

Make a Difference

As your career progresses, you will learn supervisory skills, such as processing payroll, periodic summaries, quarterly and annual returns (FUTA – Federal Unemployment Tax - 940), and other important financial forms that are associated with the practice. Remember Form W-4, which is the Employee's Withholding Allowance Certificate, must be given to new employees immediately upon hiring. The information is confidential, so it should be kept in a secure location. The W-4 should be offered to every employee at the beginning of the year in case an employee should want to change the number of allowances.

STANDARD PRECAUTIONS

NA

EQUIPMENT/SUPPLIES

Pen
Calculator
Employee Check
Wage Statement
Individual Payroll Record
Employee Information

STANDARD OF PERFORMANCE OF THE TASK

You may earn a maximum of 5 points for each competency regardless of the number of steps to be performed.

EX: If you miss two steps and achieve all the rest then you have earned 3 points.

More than five steps missed means that you have 0 points.

Your instructor may choose not to assign points but check you off on a pass or fail status.

Regardless, you may need to repeat the competency for successful completion.

It is up to your instructor to determine the maximum number of tries before the competency has been met successfully in the time allotted.

Student Name: _____   Date: _____

Time: Satisfactory   Unsatisfactory

Successful Completion: Yes   No

Grade/Points: _____   Pass   Fail

Need to Repeat: _____   Number of Attempts: 1   2   3

Instructor Comments: _____

_____

CONDITIONS UNDER WHICH THE STUDENT IS EXPECTED TO PERFORM THE TASK

Follow Task/Performance Steps

	Task/Performance Step	S	U
1.	Student enters all figures and withholdings from above to the Wage Statement form.		
2.	Student calculates the employee weekly salary by using the Wage Statement form and the information provided above.		
3.	Student transfers the calculated payroll information to the Individual Payroll Record.		
4.	Student verifies all entries for accuracy.		
5.	Student completes the payroll check to the employee using the Net Pay amount.		

Key: Satisfactory = S; Unsatisfactory = U

WAGE STATEMENT FORM

Employer _____   SS# _____

Number _____   Period From _____

Payments	No. Hours	Rate	Total
Regular Hours			
Overtime Hours			
Vacation			
		Total Earned	

KEEP THIS RECORD OF YOUR EARNINGS

Social Security (FICA)	
Federal Withholding	
State Withholding	
Local Withholding	
Insurance/Disability	
Total Deductions	
Total Net Pay	

INDIVIDUAL PAYROLL RECORD

Name _____   SS# _____

No. of Exemptions _____   Single ☐   Married ☐

	DEDUCTIONS				PAY		
Date	Social Security	Federal	State	Local	Insurance	Net Pay	Check #

Employee Payroll Check

Dr. Franklin Pierce Wright , Family Practice   **6009**
2310 Wright Way
Melbourne, FL 32904   Date _____

Pay to the
Order of _____ $ _____

_____ Dollars

Community Bank

For _____   _____

:298753098: 8624167849 3451

Part 5
Clinical Competencies

Practicum 22. Infection Control

COMPETENCY

CAAHEP: 3. b. (1) (a) Perform hand washing
ABHES: 4. (c) Apply principles of aseptic technique and infection control

SPECIFIC TASK

Perform an aseptic hand wash using the steps below within 3 minutes. Gather all supplies before the task. Hand washing is performed before and after contact with each patient, handling contaminated items, and applying pharmacology procedures.

STANDARD PRECAUTIONS

Allergies to soap, Material Safety DataSheet manual available, spillage of water on floor

EQUIPMENT/SUPPLIES

Water, liquid soap, nailbrush, or orange stick
Clean paper towels
Gloves
Proper trash receptacle

STANDARD OF PERFORMANCE OF THE TASK

You may earn a maximum of 5 points for each competency regardless of the number of steps to be performed.
   EX: If you miss two steps and achieve all the rest then you have earned 3 points
   More than five steps missed means that you have 0 points.
   Your instructor may choose not to assign points but check you off on a pass or fail status.
Regardless, you may need to repeat the competency for successful completion.
   It is up to your instructor to determine the maximum number of tries before the competency has been met successfully in the time allotted.

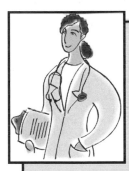

Make a Difference

Hand washing is the most effective way to help stop cross-contamination and provide infection control. With the wide spread of MRSA and VRE we must all do our part to help protect ourselves, our patients, and our communities. .Proper and frequent handwashing between each patient is the only preventative measure.

Student Name: _____ Date: _____

Time: Satisfactory   Unsatisfactory

Successful Completion: Yes   No

Grade/Points: _____   Pass   Fail

Need to Repeat: _____   Number of Attempts: 1   2   3

Instructor Comments: _____

_____

_____

CONDITIONS UNDER WHICH THE STUDENT IS EXPECTED TO PERFORM THE TASK

Follow Task/Performance Steps

Task/Performance Step	S	U
1. Gather all equipment/supplies. Make sure paper towels are available before hand washing. Make sure soap dispenser is filled.		
2. Remove all jewelry from hands and wrists. *Jewelry harbors bacteria and should not be worn during clinical performance and procedure. Wedding rings are acceptable. Wedding rings may be left on during the hand washing procedure. Place removed jewelry on a clean surface or paper towel.*		
3. Obtain paper towel. Turn the faucet on by using the paper towel, and adjust the water temperature to moderately warm.		
4. Wet both your hands thoroughly and apply a generous amount of liquid soap.		
5. Work the soap into lather making sure that all of both hands are lathered. Working with one hand at a time, interlace your fingers to clean between them, and use the palm of one hand to clean the back of the other. Rub vigorously in a circular motion for 2 minutes. *Keep your hands lower than your forearms so that the water and germs flow into the sink instead of back onto your arms. The fingertips should always be pointed down toward the sink when performing a medical aseptic hand wash. Surgical aseptic hand wash is performed with your hands pointing upward so the water runs back toward your wrist and arms.*		
6. Using the nailbrush or orange stick, dislodge the dirt around your nails and cuticles.		
7. Keeping your hands pointed toward the sink but not touching the sink or faucets, rinse your hands well.		
8. Obtain clean paper towel and dry your hands thoroughly. Discard appropriately. Using another clean paper towel turn off the faucet. Discard this paper towel appropriately.		

Key: Satisfactory = S; Unsatisfactory = U

SMART THINKING

To complete this competency, answer the following questions:

1. List 6 general pathogenic microorganisms.

_____

_____

_____

_____

2. Differentiate between direct and indirect contact.

_____

_____

_____

_____

3. Explain the difference between a medical aseptic hand wash and a surgical scrub.

_____

_____

_____

_____

Practicum 23. Telephone Screening

COMPETENCY

CAAHEP: 3. b. (4) (a) Perform telephone and in-person screening
ABHES: 4. (ff) Perform telephone and in-person screening

SPECIFIC TASK

In the time specified by your instructor, screen an incoming call from a patient requesting a refill on a BP medication.

Use a classmate to pose as the caller. Ask appropriate screening questions. Answer the phone with a greeting, your name, the office/physician name, and ask how you can assist the caller.

Your office protocol states refills on BP medication are okay to refill if the patient has been seen in the last 2 months and has had regular BP checks. You create the rest of the scenario. Document the call on the attached form.

Patient Name:	Neil Kaine
Last Seen:	16 days ago for BP check
Requested Medication:	Maxide 25 mg, takes 1/day. 30 pills.
Pharmacy:	Telephone # 934-0097. Do Good Pharmacy. (Other patient information can be obtained from the Database.)

STANDARD PRECAUTIONS

PPE, soap, and water

EQUIPMENT/SUPPLIES

Patient chart/progress note, pen, message book, phone, clock.

STANDARD OF PERFORMANCE OF THE TASK

You may earn a maximum of 5 points for each competency regardless of the number of steps to be performed.

EX: If you miss two steps and achieve all the rest then you have earned 3 points.

More than five steps missed means that you have 0 points.

Your instructor may choose not to assign points but check you off on a pass or fail status.
Regardless, you may need to repeat the competency for successful completion.

It is up to your instructor to determine the maximum number of tries before the competency has been met successfully in the time allotted.

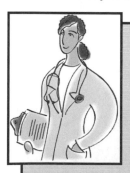

Make a Difference

You are the first impression when answering the telephone. A smile in your voice can go a long way! When screening calls, always be sure to repeat the information back. This will ensure correct information and less medical error.

Student Name: _____   Date: _____

Time: Satisfactory   Unsatisfactory

Successful Completion: Yes   No

Grade/Points: _____   Pass   Fail

Need to Repeat: _____   Number of Attempts: 1   2   3

Instructor Comments: _____

_____

_____

CONDITIONS UNDER WHICH THE STUDENT IS EXPECTED TO PERFORM THE TASK

Follow Task/Performance Steps

Task/Performance Step	S	U
1. Phone rings. Answer call within the first three rings. Have message book available and ready to write on. *Answering the phone in the first three rings gives a good first impression and shows availability.*		
2. Answer appropriately with greeting, time of day, your name, and name of practice or physician. Ask how you can assist. *This makes the patient feel important and that you are ready to assist them.*		
3. Ask the caller his/her name and phone number. Ask if caller is currently a patient of the practice. *There is always a chance that you could become disconnected, so by obtaining the number and name you can call the patient back immediately. It is not good practice to allow the patient to think they have been hung up on.*		
4. The caller will state that he requires a refill on his prescription of Maxide 25 mg. Screen the call appropriately for the correct information. *Knowing your specific office protocol with regard to refills can avoid legalities. You are an advocate of the practice and should always be informed.*		
5. Document the call in the message book. Document in the patient chart. Thorough screening includes: • Date and time call is received • Who the caller is • Caller's name and telephone number • When the caller can be reached (in case of questions) • Nature and urgency of the call • Action to be taken • Message, if any • Your name or initials (in case of questions)		
6. Repeat the information back to the caller to verify correct information. *This ensures accurate information.*		
7. Give an approximate time as to who will call the patient back, and verify the refill has been called in to the pharmacy. Document the call and action. *Do not make promises you cannot keep. When giving a time to return a call, make sure to follow through.*		

Key: Satisfactory = S; Unsatisfactory = U

MESSAGE BOOK

Name of Caller _____ Date _____ Time _____

Current Patient   Yes   No

Message For _____

Return Call _____   Caller Will Return Call _____

            Time _____   Time _____

No Call/FYI _____   Returned Your Call _____

Daytime Phone _____   Evening Phone _____

Message _____

_____

_____

Action To Be Taken _____

_____

Initials _____

PROGRESS NOTE – DOCUMENTATION

Name Student/Patient _____

DOB _____

Allergies _____

Date _____

_____

_____

_____

Instructor Corrections _____

_____

_____

_____

Practicum 24. Vital Signs

COMPETENCY

CAAHEP: 3. b. (4) (b) Obtain vital signs
           3. c. (2) (e) Document appropriately
ABHES: 4. (d) Take vital signs
           5. (b) Document accurately

SPECIFIC TASK

This competency will challenge you but will also allow you to focus on your multitasking skills. This competency is set up in this fashion because during your externship and employment you will find you generally take all the vitals signs together. You will manage your assessment time easier if you take your vitals in the correct order.

In the time specified by your instructor, obtain a height, weight, temperature, BP, pulse, and respiration from a classmate posing as the patient. Count the pulse and respiration for 1 full minute before determining the rate. Document your results.

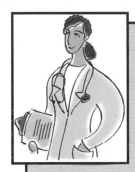

Make a Difference

Counting pulse and respiration for 1 full minute when first learning the skill helps you to identify and learn the different characteristics of the pulse and respiration. For a pulse, you should document the rate as well as the rhythm and pulse volume. For respiration, you should document the rate as well as the rhythm and depth. By performing these tasks for 1 full minute, you will learn to identify the different sounds and depths. Once you have fully learned how to identify all characteristics, it will be easier for you to distinguish when you are multiplying your rates to save time.

STANDARD PRECAUTIONS

PPE, soap, and water

EQUIPMENT/SUPPLIES

Black pen/red pen
Progress note/chart
Sphygmomanometer/stethoscope
Watch with a second hand
Calibrated height/weight scale
Paper towels
Thermometer (types may vary, use what instructor has assigned)

STANDARD OF PERFORMANCE OF THE TASK

You may earn a maximum of 5 points for each competency regardless of the number of steps to be performed.

EX: If you miss two steps and achieve all the rest then you have earned 3 points.

More than five steps missed means that you have 0 points.

Your instructor may choose not to assign points but check you off on a pass or fail status. Regardless, you may need to repeat the competency for successful completion.

It is up to your instructor to determine the maximum number of tries before the competency has been met successfully in the time allotted.

Student Name: _____   Date: _____

Time: Satisfactory   Unsatisfactory

Successful Completion: Yes   No

Grade/Points: _____   Pass   Fail

Need to Repeat: _____   Number of Attempts: 1   2   3

Instructor Comments: _____

_____

_____

CONDITIONS UNDER WHICH THE STUDENT IS EXPECTED TO PERFORM THE TASK

Follow Task/Performance Steps

Task/Performance Step	S	U
HEIGHT/WEIGHT		
1. Identify and greet the patient. Identify yourself. Explain the procedure. On the way to the examination room/table, stop and take the Height and Weight.		
2. Preplace a paper towel on the scale where the feet will stand. Balance the scale by assuring that both 50 lb and sliding pound bar weights are on zero and that the pointed end of bar is floating in the middle of the balance frame. *Using a paper towel helps prevent cross-contamination. Always be consistent when taking height and weight to ensure patient record and vital consistency. Always take height and weight with shoes on or shoes off. Check to see what your physician preference is.*		
3. Have the patient take off his/her shoes and any other heavy objects and set them aside.		
4. Lift height bar and raise higher than the patient's head. Assist the patient on the scale with their back toward the scale so that he/she is facing you. Steady the patient by offering your arm. *Elderly and younger patients may need more assistance. Always watch that they are steady so as not to tip the scale or fall off. This helps to prevent liabilities.*		
5. Gently lower the height bar at the point of measurement (top of patient's head). Leave the height bar at the point of measurement.		
6. Move the larger weight to the nearest approximate 50 lb weight notch, increase to the next if necessary. Move the smaller weight to the number at which the bar floats in the middle of the balance frame.		
7. Protect the patient's head and have them step down. *Always offer a helping hand.*		
8. Add weight measurements to the nearest 0.25 lb. Take height measurement to the nearest 0.25 in.		
9. Instruct patient to put on their shoes and gather any belongings. Discard the paper towel appropriately. Thank the patient.		
10. Immediately record the results in the patient chart while walking the patient to the examination room where it is quiet, comfortable, and private.		

TEMPERATURE		
1. Ask the patient if he/she has had anything to eat or drink or smoked in the last 15 minutes. Ask if they have anything in their mouth that does not belong. *Items such as dentures or other orthotic devices are mostly made of porcelain and hard plastic and can cause some thermometers to break. Ask the patient not to bite down on the thermometer and to try to breathe through the nose. Be sure the patient keeps their mouth closed until you have removed the thermometer.*		
2. If the patient did not eat, drink, or smoke and you are taking an oral temperature you may continue, otherwise wait for 15 minutes and then continue.		
3. If you are using a glass oral thermometer, hold the thermometer into the light and check for any cracks or breaks.		
4. If you are using a glass, mercury, oral thermometer, hold with a firm grip and away from furniture or the patient; firmly shake with a quick hard downward motion 2–3 times until the mercury reaches 96.0 degrees. If you are using any other type of thermometer, prepare as the manufacturer suggests.		
5. Insert the thermometer into the sheath covering if applicable. Insert the thermometer under the tongue or appropriate site. Wait the allotted time according to the equipment you are using (three minutes for oral temperature). *It is best to take temperature first and then start other vitals, especially if you are taking an oral temperature that takes 3 minutes. This way you use time wisely.*		
6. After 3 minutes or allotted time, remove the thermometer and note the result. Document the temperature. Wash hands.		
BLOOD PRESSURE, PULSE, AND RESPIRATION		
1. Perform medical aseptic hand wash. *Prevents cross-contamination from patient to patient.*		
2. Gather all necessary equipment, a black and red pen, and the patient record. *The chart/progress note or record is a legal document. Only use black ink. The red pen is for addressing any allergies to the patient only.*		
3. Introduce and identify yourself, then identify the patient. Escort the patient to the examination room. *If you smile, the patient will enjoy a friendly atmosphere.*		
4. Vitals will be more accurate if the patient is sitting with legs uncrossed.		
5. Instruct the patient about the procedure. Inform the patient you will be taking his/her BP and pulse. *When assessing respiration, the patient should breathe naturally; therefore, never inform the patient that you will be taking the respiration.*		
6. Palpate the brachial artery in the left arm while supporting the patient's arm between your arm and side. *Using the left arm and offering support so that the patient is not just holding the arm or wrist out dangling will support a more accurate reading for both the physician and the patient.*		
7. Wrap the cuff snuggly around the patient's arm staying about 1 inch above the natural crease of the elbow with the BP bladder over the brachial artery. *Inform the patient that the cuff will get tight but you will immediately release the pressure. This ensures cooperation from the patient and stops any alarm that the patient may have when the cuff is inflated.*		
8. Determine maximum inflation level by palpating the radial pulse and inflating cuff until pulse is no longer felt. Deflate cuff while mentally adding 30 to the number registered when the pulse was obliterated. Inflate cuff and read pressure.		
9. Wait 1–2 minutes and then take the patient's pulse.		
10. Still supporting the patient's left arm, gently lay the arm and hand on examination table or the patient's lap. Explain you will now take a pulse.		

	By supporting the left limb, you will not create a value from exertion of lifting. Too often the patient holds the arm out for you. This will increase the BP and the pulse rate.		
11.	Gently compress the radial artery against the radius with tips of the first two or three fingers. Be sure to feel the pulse. Count for 1 full minute. *In the beginning, you should always count 1 full minute to hear for irregularities in the pulse. After you have mastered the skill you can count palpations for 30 seconds and multiply by two.*		
12.	While counting, remember to assess the rhythm and strength of the pulse for documentation.		
13.	Once you have mentally recorded the pulse rate, obtain the respiration rate. *You do not want your patient to know that you are counting the number of breaths, so continue to look as though you are counting the pulse by keeping your hand and finger on the wrist.*		
14.	Count each rise and fall of the chest for 1 full minute. *One full inspiration and one full expiration make one respiration. Be sure to note the rhythm and depth of the respiration as well as the rate. Prior assessment of your patient will help you identify any bulky clothing that may inhibit your view of the chest. If this is the case, the clothing items can be removed and/or a patient gown can be used.*		
15.	Document the pulse and respiration.		
16.	Check your stethoscope to make sure you hear audible sounds. *Too many times your stethoscope could accidentally be turned off or becomes inaudible.*		
17.	Place the diaphragm of the stethoscope on the artery firmly enough to seal but lightly enough to avoid obliterating the artery. *Tubing that rubs together or touches the scope itself can create false sounds. Make sure your tubing is not crossed with the cuff, and you will hear the BP much easier.*		
18.	Close the valve with your thumb using a right turn motion..		
19.	Squeeze bulb and inflate cuff in a rapid smooth motion. *Another helpful tip is to ask the patient if the previous blood pressure was known or if he/she knows what it runs normally. You can look in the chart for a previous reading. This will help you determine how high to inflate the cuff so an accurate reading is obtained.*		
20.	Open the valve just slightly to deflate the cuff at about 2 mm per second, watching the gauge and listening for the first distinct sound. Remember this number. *The first sound is the systolic reading.*		
21.	Continue listening until the last distinct sound appears. Remember this number. *The last distinct sound is the Diastolic reading.*		
22.	Open the valve and deflate the cuff all the way. Remove the cuff and replace the sphygmomanometer in the holder or pouch.		
23.	Thank the patient. Restate your name and offer any additional assistance or that you would be happy to answer any questions. Let the patient know the physician will be there as soon as he can. *Know your office protocol before supplying vital results to the patient.*		
24.	Wash your hands. *Washing your hands first, before documenting; helps prevent cross-contamination from the chart or progress note.*		
25.	Document the results. Wash your hands. *The uses of nursing symbols have changed. Be aware of your documentation.*		

Key: Satisfactory = S; Unsatisfactory = U

SMART THINKING

Answer the following questions using the space provided. Some research may be necessary to answer correctly.

1. Look around your laboratory or use reference books or the Internet, and name at least four different types of thermometers.

_____

_____

2. What are the normal values for the following?

a. Oral T – _____

b. Rectal T – _____

c. Axillary T – _____

3. What is "dyspnea"?

_____

_____

4. What is the pulse pressure for a patient with a BP of 180/84? Is this normal or abnormal?

_____

PROGRESS NOTE – DOCUMENTATION

Name Student/Patient _____

DOB _____

Allergies _____

Date _____

HT _____   WT _____

T _____   BP _____   P _____   R _____

_____

Instructor Corrections/Comments _____

_____

_____

Practicum 25. Patient History/Communication

COMPETENCY

CAAHEP: 3. b. (4) (c) Obtain and record patient history
3. c. (1) (b) Recognize and respond to verbal communication
3. c. (1) (c) Recognize and respond to nonverbal communication

ABHES: 2. (a) Be attentive, listen, and learn
2. (f) Interview effectively
2. (i) Recognize and respond to verbal and nonverbal communication
2. (j) Use correct grammar, spelling, and formatting techniques in written works
2. (k) Principles of verbal and nonverbal communication
2. (l) Recognition and response to verbal and nonverbal communication
4. (a) Interview and take a patient history

SPECIFIC TASK

In the time specified by your instructor, use a classmate as your patient and obtain and record a patient history using interviewing technique. Be attentive and listen for verbal and nonverbal feedback. Recognize and respond as the questions are asked and answered. For documentation purposes, use the form provided. Apply written words using the format already provided in the form. Check your work for grammar and spelling.

Taking vital signs is optional and at the discretion of your instructor.

PATIENT: MARCUS PLAN

Current Medications: Lasix 10 mg 1/day, Lipitor 10 mg 1/day, nitroglycerin PRN (Refer to Database.)

During the history interview you notice that Mr. Plan keeps clenching his fists and grabbing the left upper quadrant of his chest. You also witness the look of discomfort in his face during this time (nonverbal communication).

You question him several times and he states nothing is wrong. Near the end of the history he finally admits he is in great discomfort. Be sure to encourage Mr. Plan to speak freely and let him know that all information will be kept confidential but that open communication will help facilitate how the physician will help him further. You recognize both the verbal and nonverbal communication and respond by assuring Mr. Plan that the physician will first address his discomfort (verbal communication).

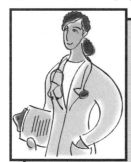

Make a Difference

Practicing vitals as much as you can will strengthen your ability to get accurate results. Assessing your patient by carefully observing the verbal and nonverbal language will aid you in asking appropriate questions and interpreting the answers. By the time you are ready for your externship you will have mastered the skill.

Good assessment skills come from actively listening to your patient and recognizing nonverbal communication. As a physician's assistant, you will obtain the history by interviewing the patient. Although the physician performs the physical portion of the History and Physical, you will often assist the physician with the documentation, the physical examination, or diagnostic tests that have been ordered, so it is good practice to be able to identify any special terminology that may be used when reviewing or actually examining the Review of Systems.

STANDARD PRECAUTIONS

PPE, soap, and water

EQUIPMENT/SUPPLIES

History and physical form provided
Black and red ink pen
Optional: If vitals are taken
Sphygmomanometer
Stethoscope
Watch/second hand

STANDARD OF PERFORMANCE OF THE TASK

You may earn a maximum of 5 points for each competency regardless of the number of steps to be performed.

EX: If you miss two steps and achieve all the rest then you have earned 3 points.

More than five steps missed means that you have 0 points.

Your instructor may choose not to assign points but check you off on a pass or fail status.

Regardless, you may need to repeat the competency for successful completion.

It is up to your instructor to determine the maximum number of tries before the competency has been met successfully in the time allotted.

Student Name: _____ Date: _____

Time: Satisfactory   Unsatisfactory

Successful Completion: Yes   No

Grade/Points: _____   Pass   Fail

Need to Repeat: _____   Number of Attempts: 1   2   3

Instructor Comments: _____

_____

_____

CONDITIONS UNDER WHICH THE STUDENT IS EXPECTED TO PERFORM THE TASK

Follow Task/Performance Steps

Task/Performance Step	S	U
1. Greet and identify the patient. Identify and introduce yourself. *Ensures you have the "Right Patient." By introducing yourself, the patient can also call you by your name.*		
2. Explain the procedure. Assure the patient that he/she can ask you questions, too. *One question generally leads to another. When a patient asks a question back, it may lead you to another topic and will then provide for a more thorough history.*		
3. Gather necessary supplies and equipment. Perform a medical aseptic hand wash. *Gathering supplies ahead of time is a good time management skill. Hand washing prevents cross-contamination even if just handling documents. Everyone handles paperwork. You cannot be certain that others are adhering to standards. Washing your hands frequently will keep you and the environment safer.*		
4. When or if you are performing vitals, refer to competency b4b or 4a. *This is a skill you have already mastered. Practice makes perfect!*		
5. Using the history form provided, begin to assess your patient by asking the appropriate questions. Remember you have noted nonverbal communication, which should be documented. *Watch the patient (classmate) for any other nonverbal signs of communication. Follow through with verbal communication.*		
6. During documentation, use as many symbols and abbreviations as allowed. Use only those that are approved and legal. Nursing symbols have changed. *Always remember to only give the physician the facts and what the patient states making sure you are capturing the entire SOAP format.*		
7. After properly assessing and documenting, ask the patient if there are any questions or concerns to further facilitate communication and understanding. *This helps to alleviate anxieties the patient may have. The patient's questions may give you more information that will assist the physician in the H&P process, which in turn makes the patient feel like his/her own advocate in health care.*		
8. Thank the patient. *This helps to build a professional, trusting relationship for future visits.*		
9. Wash your hands. Review your documentation. *Normally the chart is put outside the examination room door in a specific area where the physician can review it before seeing the patient.*		

Key: Satisfactory = S; Unsatisfactory = U

HISTORY/PHYSICAL FORM

Name Student/Patient _____

DOB _____

Allergies _____

Date _____

Pt states reason for visit _____

_____

HT _____ WT _____

T _____ BP _____ P _____ R _____

Current Medications _____

Demographic _____

_____

SH (Social History) _____

_____

FH (Family History) _____

_____

Relative _____ Living _____ DC _____ Age _____

Cause of Death _____

Relative _____ Living _____ DC _____ Age _____

Cause of Death _____

PMH (Prior Medical History)
Surgeries _____

Hospitalization _____

Adult Immunizations _____

Childhood Immunizations _____

PI (Present Illness) _____

SP (Self Perception) _____

PE (Physical Examination)
ROS (Review of Systems) _____

HEENT _____

Respiratory _____

_____

Urinary _____

_____

Gastrointestinal _____

_____

Reproductive _____

_____

Musculoskeletal _____

_____

Integumentary _____

_____

Neurological _____

_____

Assessment _____

_____

Treatment/Plan _____

_____

_____

SMART THINKING

Define the following acronyms.

HEENT _____

PEERLA _____

PEARL _____

WNL _____

Practicum 26. Examination and Treatment Areas

COMPETENCY

CAAHEP: 3. b. (4) (d) Prepare and maintain examination and treatment areas
ABHES: 1. (c) Be a "team player"
          1. (e) Exhibit initiative
          4. (g) Prepare and maintain examination and treatment areas

SPECIFIC TASK

Your instructor will or already has assigned an "examination room station, or table, or area in the laboratory or classroom" in which you are responsible for preparation, reporting, maintenance, lighting, ventilation, stocking of supplies and equipment, adhering to safety, and disinfecting any areas that require it due to bloodborne pathogens. As an example of some daily tasks, your examination rooms should be disinfected daily, and the lighting should be reported if you feel there is a malfunction. The examination table should be covered with clean paper, and all evidence of previous patients should be removed.

Your assigned station will be viewed and inspected by your instructor throughout the semester/module to ensure you are following proper protocol and adhering to the procedure manual (Database). Each time you perform a task, document the task in the form provided below. You should document that you maintained your examination and treatment area 10 times. When you have completed your assigned duties, your instructor will check you off. You will demonstrate initiative by helping a classmate with their assigned duties without being asked. This shows "team effort" and you end up helping each other.

STANDARD PRECAUTIONS

PPE, soap, water, and gloves

EQUIPMENT/SUPPLIES

All daily medical supplies that you would find in an examination/laboratory room. Access to stock supplies. Table paper and disinfectant. Supplies may vary on this competency, and are up to your instructor.

STANDARD OF PERFORMANCE OF THE TASK

You may earn a maximum of 5 points for each competency regardless of the number of steps to be performed.

EX: If you miss two steps and achieve all the rest then you have earned 3 points.

More than five steps missed means that you have 0 points.

Your instructor may choose not to assign points but check you off on a pass or fail status.
Regardless, you may need to repeat the competency for successful completion.

It is up to your instructor to determine the maximum number of tries before the competency has been met successfully in the time allotted.

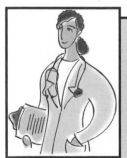

Make a Difference

Maintenance, stocking, and keeping a clean workplace environment are essential to the safety and success of any practice. Knowing your daily procedure/maintenance schedule will allow you to work in a hazard free and safer workplace. Showing initiative demonstrates you can be a team player.

Student Name: _____ Date: _____

Time:	Satisfactory	Unsatisfactory
Successful Completion:	Yes	No
Grade/Points: _____	Pass	Fail

Need to Repeat: _____ Number of Attempts: 1 2 3

Instructor Comments: _____

_____

_____

CONDITIONS UNDER WHICH THE STUDENT IS EXPECTED TO PERFORM THE TASK

Follow Task/Performance Steps

Task/Performance Step	S	U
1. Obtain office procedure manual and follow instructions for daily, monthly, and yearly maintenance of examination rooms and workplace. *The office procedural manual gives you explanation on what is expected of maintenance of examination and treatment areas.*		
2. Gather all appropriate supplies and/or disinfectants to complete the task.		
3. Inform the instructor your station has been maintained. *Allows the instructor to ensure the station or your assigned duty has been maintained nearly every class day properly. By actively taking a role in your station here, you will automatically be reminded what to do upon employment. The instructor will initial the date and task performed.*		
4. Adhered to assigned duties/station regularly.		
5. Completed assignment in a timely fashion.		
6. Student exhibited initiative by assisting a fellow classmate.		

Key: Satisfactory = S; Unsatisfactory = U

MAINTENANCE OF EXAMINATION AND TREATMENT AREA DOCUMENTATION

Date	Task Completed	Instructor Initials

Date	Task Completed	Instructor Initials

INITIATIVE/TEAM PLAYER

Date	Task Completed/For	Instructor Initials

Practicum 27. Assisting With Examinations

COMPETENCY

CAAHEP: 3. b. (4) (e) Prepare patient for and assist with routine and specialty examinations
          3. b. (2) (e) Instruct patients in the collection of fecal specimens
ABHES: 2. (b) Be impartial and show empathy when dealing with patients
          2. (g) Use appropriate medical terminology
          4. (h) Assist physician with examinations and treatments
          4. (k) Perform selected tests that assist with diagnosis and treatment
          4. (x) Instruct patient in the collection of fecal specimen

SPECIFIC TASK

In the time specified by your instructor, prepare a patient for a routine PAP Smear Examination and obtain a gynecological history. This task will require draping and positioning the patient properly and assembling the appropriate equipment and supplies. Your instructor or classmates can role-play as the physician. You will assist the physician during the examination.

   This physician will also require an occult stool specimen during the PAP examination. You will document that the occult stool test was positive. The physician requests that you instruct the patient to collect a fecal specimen at home using the brand your program/laboratory supplies. You will follow manufacturer instructions for obtaining the specimen from the patient.

   Patient Name: Debby Verisso
   Information: Database

STANDARD PRECAUTIONS

PPE, soap, water, mask, gloves, gown

EQUIPMENT/SUPPLIES

Gloves, disinfectant, soap and water, biohazard container, lubricating gel, vaginal speculum, light source, gauze, vaginal/cervical scraper, occult blood test and developer, glass slide for samples or wet preparation, fixative spray, laboratory requisition form, biohazard transportation bag, stool for the physician to sit on, drape and gown for patient, and patient progress note.

STANDARD OF PERFORMANCE OF THE TASK

You may earn a maximum of 5 points for each competency regardless of the number of steps to be performed.
   EX: If you miss two steps and achieve all the rest then you have earned 3 points.
   More than five steps missed means that you have 0 points.
   Your instructor may choose not to assign points but check you off on a pass or fail status.
Regardless, you may need to repeat the competency for successful completion.
   It is up to your instructor to determine the maximum number of tries before the competency has been met successfully in the time allotted.

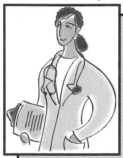

Make a Difference

Assisting the physician with treatment and diagnostic tests is a serious responsibility. Always read the manufacturer's instructions and follow all quality assurance/control steps before actually performing the test for patient results. Remember to document your results accurately, and bring the results to the attention of the physician.

Student Name: _____   Date: _____

Time: Satisfactory   Unsatisfactory

Successful Completion: Yes   No

Grade/Points: _____   Pass   Fail

Need to Repeat: _____   Number of Attempts: 1   2   3

Instructor Comments: _____

_____

_____

CONDITIONS UNDER WHICH THE STUDENT IS EXPECTED TO PERFORM THE TASK

Follow Task/Performance Steps

Task/Performance Step	S	U
1. Gather and assemble equipment and supplies. Ready the examination room for the patient. Be sure to cover the PAP tray so it is not noticeable to the patient upon entering the room. *By checking the appointment book ahead of time, you can manage your time and be prepared for all examinations, treatments, or tests that require prior set up. Always try to stay a few steps ahead of the physician.*		
2. Perform aseptic hand wash. *Helps to stop cross-contamination from any fomites that you might have touched during set up.*		
3. Greet the patient, identify yourself, and confirm the patient's identity adhering to HIPAA. Escort the patient to the examination room. *The Right Patient is important. Adhering to HIPAA privacy says you call by the first name and ask the last name in a private area.*		
4. Document the gynecological history on the form provided below. Note the special medical terminology. Research the terms if you are not familiar before you take the history. *Remember subjective + objective information assists the physician in his assessment.*		
5. Explain the procedure to the patient, and advise them to put on the gown with the opening in the front. Provide privacy and let her know you will return shortly. *Good patient instructions will earn cooperation from the patient. Courtesy says check the temperature of the room and offer a blanket if necessary. Let the patient know where to lay her clothes. No one likes this examination. By doing the little things that count, you will give the act of impartiality and empathy to the situation.*		
6. Knock before entering the room and identify yourself at the same time. *Courtesy and empathy to the patient in case they are still in the middle of changing. Surprises are best left for birthdays!*		
7. Wrap a warm towel over the stirrups or use the disposable foot covers. Paper towels are a nice substitute. *Stirrups can be cold on the feet and the cover harbors bacteria from too many feet. Always disinfect the feet stirrups. Show you care by using a stirrup cover.*		

EMPATHY		
8. Assist the patient in the Lithotomy position. Drape point to chin. *For patients who are not limber enough for the lithotomy position, use the alternate position. You may need to assist some patients.*		
9. Check your light source and let the physician know you are ready.		
10. While assisting the physician, talk to the patient to help ease the examination process. This helps show empathy for the "position" they are in!		
11. Put on your gloves. Assist the physician with his. *The physician will require two gloves to start and then a clean glove for the rectal/occult blood examination.*		
12. Pull back the point of the drape just enough to expose the area for the physician.		
13. Hand the physician the vaginal speculum and 4x4 gauze with the lubricant gel. He will lubricate the vaginal speculum for insertion. *How and when the physician lubricates the speculum is office/physician protocol. Some may wish for it to be prelubed before the physician coming into the room.*		
14. First, hand the physician the vaginal/cervical scraper with the vaginal side first. The physician will collect the specimen, so have the slide or wet preparation ready. *Reminder: Some physicians will take an endocervical specimen as well, so have the endo brush ready to hand the physician as well as the slide. If using a slide, it should be clearly marked with a C, V, and E.*		
15. After the specimens have been collected, spray a generous amount of fixative spray directly on the slide or cap the wet prep. The physician will remove the speculum. Be prepared to take it and set it on the tray. *By spraying fixative, the specimen is secured to the slide for transportation to the laboratory. You will need to complete a cytology requisition form. It is better to already have the form prepared ahead of time and have it in the transport bag. This will help prevent cross-contamination.*		
16. The physician will remove one glove from his dominant hand for a new one to perform the bimanual examination. Don the new glove on the physician. *This will be office/physician protocol. Some physicians may or may not perform the bimanual examination. An occult stool test card should be available to apply the stool specimen.*		
17. Hold the occult stool test card so the physician can apply the stool specimen. Apply the proper amount of drops and read the test result. You will document this one positive. *Be sure to address the result with the physician for further instructions. Record the results.*		
18. Cover the tray until the patient has been taken care of. Offer tissue or a method of cleaning after the examination. Tell her she may dress, where to place the gown and tissue, and that you will give her privacy and return momentarily. Remove your gloves and wash hands. *This ensures patient privacy and common courtesy.*		
19. Knock before entering. Instruct the patient in the collection of the fecal specimen according to the type of tests you have available and when to return to the clinic. Ask the patient if there are any questions. Escort the patient to the reception area. Thank the patient.		
20. Return to the examination room. Put on clean gloves. Tear down the tray and clean the examination room according to OSHA standards. Document.		

Key: Satisfactory = S; Unsatisfactory = U

PROGRESS NOTE – DOCUMENTATION

Name Student/Patient _____

DOB _____

Allergies _____

_____

_____

_____

_____

GYNECOLOGICAL HISTORY QUESTIONNAIRE

Date of last menstrual period _____

Cycle _____

Date of last PAP _____

Gravida _____

Para _____

Gynecological Surgery _____

Radiation Therapy _____

Lab to _____

Instructor Corrections _____

_____

_____

_____

SMART THINKING

Provide the definition for the following terms or acronyms.

Braxton Hicks _____

Goodell's Sign _____

Chadwick's Sign _____

Primigravida _____

Secundigravida _____

Nulligravida _____

EDC _____

EDD _____

VDRL _____

RPR _____

Ectopic Pregnancy _____

Endometritis _____

Practicum 28. Assisting with Procedures

COMPETENCY

CAAHEP: 3. b. (4) (f) Prepare patient for and assist with procedures, treatments, and minor office
                surgery
            3. b. (1) (b) Wrap items for autoclaving
            3. b. (1) (c) Perform sterilization techniques

ABHES: 4. (b) Prepare patients for procedures
            4. (o) Wrap items for autoclaving
            4. (p) Perform sterilization techniques

SPECIFIC TASK

Your instructor will assign instruments and the type of autoclaving materials that will be used in the competency.

Before the sterilization (autoclaving) of any instruments, they should always be scrubbed in a sink first and then soaked in the instrument lubricant for 5 minutes.

Wrap or bag your assigned instruments along with six pieces of 4x4 gauze and use a kit preparing these items for sterilization in the autoclave using the steps below. These instruments can be used to perform the minor surgery or your instructor may assign a surgical kit.

Your patient presents with a sebaceous cyst on the left posterior portion of the upper arm (deltoid area), and the physician has asked you to prepare and assist with a minor surgery. Gather and assemble all necessary items, including any patient education materials, all within the time specified by your instructor.

Assist the physician (instructor) or (classmate) with the minor surgery, handing all necessary instruments and supplies while maintaining the sterile field. You will role-play the postop care of the patient, providing any special instructions. Follow manufacturer's instructions if you are using a surgical prepared kit.

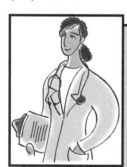

Make a Difference

Surgical asepsis prevents microorganisms from entering the body. Adhering to surgical asepsis for sterile procedures is a must to prevent infection. Accidents happen, but honesty is the best policy if you should ever break a sterile field or contaminate an item. Admit your mistake immediately to the physician. The physician will respect your honesty in the long run and you will feel better about admitting your error.

STANDARD PRECAUTIONS

PPE, sterile surgical gloves, gowns, masks, booties, bouffant cap, biohazard container, sharps container, and disinfectant
MSDS manual available for chemicals
First aid for steam or moist heat burns
Strong, durable utility gloves.

EQUIPMENT/SUPPLIES

The supplies will vary depending on availability in your classroom/laboratory
The instructor may choose to improvise on some supplies
Surgical gloves for you and the physician, surgical tray, Iris Scissors, Mayo-Hegar Needle holders, hemostats, #15 scalpel (disposable or stainless) with handle, Thumb Forceps, 3.0 Chromic and 6.0 Nylon suture material, formalin bottle for transport of specimen, sterile gauze, surgical scrub and solution for preparation, fenestrated drape, 2–4 operating room (OR) towels, 4 towel clamps, lidocaine 2% with epinephrine for local anesthetic, two 27 G needles, alcohol preps or cotton and alcohol, sterile water for irrigation and clean up, two 3 cc syringes, surgical skin marker, measuring tool, and laboratory requisition form.
Instant sealing pouches, paper, muslin, gauze, OR towel wrap.
Dry, sanitized, lubricated instruments, sterilization indicators or autoclave tape or black nonsoluble marker, large bowl for soaking instruments, autoclave and autoclave trays, instrument cleaner/lubricant, instrument brush/bottle cleaner, two dry towels, oven mitt, sterile transfer forceps

STANDARD OF PERFORMANCE OF THE TASK

You may earn a maximum of 5 points for each competency regardless of the number of steps to be performed.
    EX: If you miss two steps and achieve all the rest then you have earned 3 points.
    More than five steps missed means that you have 0 points.
    Your instructor may choose not to assign points but check you off on a pass or fail status.
Regardless, you may need to repeat the competency for successful completion.
    It is up to your instructor to determine the maximum number of tries before the competency has been met successfully in the time allotted.

Student Name: _____   Date: _____

Time: Satisfactory   Unsatisfactory

Successful Completion: Yes   No

Grade/Points: _____   Pass   Fail

Need to Repeat: _____   Number of Attempts: 1   2   3

Instructor Comments: _____

_____

_____

CONDITIONS UNDER WHICH THE STUDENT IS EXPECTED TO PERFORM THE TASK

Follow Task/Performance Steps

Task/Performance Step	S	U
WRAP ITEMS FOR AUTOCLAVING AND PERFORM STERILIZATION TECHNIQUES		
1. Gather all necessary items and prepare lubricant solution. Perform aseptic hand wash and put on utility gloves.		
2. Turn on water in sink and let run until warm. Place instruments in sink under warm running water. With brush, scrub instrument front and back. Open instruments and scrub interlocking components or serrated edge or teeth carefully with instrument cleaner. Rinse instruments.		
3. Place instruments on clean dry towel. Pat dry. Place instruments in lubricant and allow soaking for 5 minutes.		
4. Carefully remove instruments and place on towel to dry.		
5. Remove utility gloves and store in proper place. Perform aseptic hand wash.		
6. Put on regular latex gloves for handling instruments.		
IF USING AN INSTANT SEALING POUCH:		
7. Obtain correct size instant sealing pouch and label what the contents will be, the date of sterilization, and your initials in the appropriate place. *Some instruments come with manufacturer's directions. Needles and some instruments will need to be placed into special holders inside the pouch.*		
8. Inspect each item to make sure it is operating correctly. Insert the items into the pouch. Wrap any sharp ends with gauze to prevent puncturing the pouch and to protect the ends of the instruments. *All handles must be facing the end that opens after sterilization. Hinged items should be placed in the open position.*		
9. Most pouches have sterilization indicators built in to the pouch. If not, insert your indicator and check it to make sure it is not damaged or it has not already been exposed. Close and seal the pouch.		
10. Put the pack aside until you are ready to load the autoclave chamber.		
11. Remove your gloves, dispose of them in the proper waste container, and wash your hands.		
IF USING PAPER, FABRIC, OR MUSLIN:		
12. Perform aseptic hand wash and put on gloves.		
13. Place the material square on a flat surface with one point toward you. The material must be large enough for the four points to cover the instruments or equipment and provide an overlap.		

14. Always place gauze under instruments in the center of your diamond along with your instruments. *Items that will be used together can be packed together. All handles and points should be facing the same way.*		
15. Place the sterilization indicator inside the pack, and position it according to the manufacturer's guidelines or use the autoclave tape, which is also a sterilization indicator.		
16. Place each item being wrapped in the center of the pack. Fold the bottom of the diamond up and over the instruments and into the center. Fold back a small portion of the point to use later as the nonsterile area to open the sterile pack. You may refer to pictures in any textbook for exact folds.		
17. Fold the right point of the diamond into the center. Again, fold back a small portion of the point to be used later as a nonsterile area. Continue the same with the left point.		
18. Take the remaining point (your pack should look like an envelope now) and fold this portion up, toward the top point. Fold the top point down over the pack, making sure the pack is snug but not too tight.		
19. Close the pack with autoclave tape. Be sure to place a tabby folding a small portion of the tape under itself at the opening end of the tape for ease of opening later.		
20. Label the pack with your initials, the contents, and the date. You can write directly on the tape. *If pack contains items pertaining to size, indicate the size.*		
21. Put the pack aside for loading the autoclave. Remove gloves and wash hands.		
PERFORM STERILIZATION USING THE AUTOCLAVE.		
22. Check autoclave and make sure plug is connected. Check the water reservoir and fill to desired level if necessary. Check autoclave chamber for items left before you use it.		
23. Wash your hands and put on gloves.		
24. Check water level on the bottom of the chamber and fill to line. Insert packs and pouches on their sides to allow for adequate steam to flow between them. *Do not overload the chamber of an autoclave. Jars and separate containers should be placed on their sides with the lids sterile-side down.*		
25. If your load contains both wrapped packs and individual instruments, place the tray containing the instruments below the tray containing the wrapped packs.		
26. Start the timer so the desired temperature and pressure can be reached. *There are three variables in the sterilizing cycle of an autoclave: time, temperature, and pressure. Fifteen minutes at 250 degrees is adequate time to kill all known microorganisms, but times will vary depending on the load.*		
27. Once the desired temperature has been reached, reset the timer for the actual cycle of sterilization.		
28. Once the autoclave timer has sounded, vent the chamber to release all the pressure.		
29. Some autoclaves have an automatic drying cycle. Listen for the ringer to sound.		
30. With your oven mitt and standing a fair distance from the chamber, pull the handle and allow the door to swing open and the steam to escape. *Steam is hot and will burn you. Keep your distance and handle the door and objects with care. Safety first!*		
31. Once the manual or automatic drying cycle is complete, with the oven mitt on, remove the items from the chamber. Use transfer forceps for individual items.		
32. Allow items to dry in an area that is not overly cool. Check each package or item for moisture on the wrapping, underexposed sterilization indicators, and tears in the wrapping. These items are considered unsterile.		
33. Remove gloves, dispose of them in the proper waste container, and wash your hands.		

PREPARE PATIENT FOR AND ASSIST WITH PROCEDURES, TREATMENTS, AND MINOR OFFICE SURGERY		
1. Wash hands and gather all necessary equipment and supplies. *A responsible practitioner is always prepared. Check all equipment and supplies ahead of time for function. Laboratory requisition forms, formalin, preop and postop supplies should be ready in advance.*		
2. Assemble the surgical tray according to sterile technique. You may use a classmate as a circulator to assist you with sterile items. Ready the room for the patient. The tray should not be visible to the patient. Cover with a sterile towel. *The circulator will hand you sterile items to open onto the sterile tray. You will need to perform surgical aseptic hand wash and don sterile gloves and apparel. Remember sterile to sterile and unsterile to unsterile.*		
3. Call the patient. Identify yourself to the patient. Explain the procedure. *Remember to always double-check the chart for history of high BP, potential allergies, or contraindications. It is too late once the surgery begins!*		
4. Properly position the patient on the surgical/examination table in the supine position. Explain what you are doing as you go along. Prep the skin with the scrub and solution and apply the fenestrated drape and OR towels with towel clamps. *If you are touching anything sterile, you should also be sterile. The circulator is not sterile and can perform the preparation if you are already sterile.*		
5. Remind the patient you have created a sterile field and to remain still.		
6. Let the physician know you are ready to begin. The physician will be scrubbing while you have prepped the patient.		
7. Assemble 27-G needle to 3-cc syringe and hand to physician. Lift the anesthetic solution, and the physician will insert the needle and withdraw desired amount. *Be prepared to blot the local anesthetic site.*		
8. After the physician determines the site is numb, hand over the #15 blade for incision of skin. Again, be prepared to blot. *It is imperative that the physician is able to see the surgical site once the incision has been made. The blood must be kept dry.*		
9. The physician will ask for instruments as he excises the cyst, so be prepared to hand instruments and blot at the same time. *Coordination is the key to assisting the physician during surgery. Always be one step ahead of the physician. Keeping the tray organized is good quality assurance.*		
10. Talk to your patient during the surgery. *Allows courtesy and compassion and helps you to identify verbal and nonverbal language during the procedure. Always check the patient for signs of distress.*		
11. Once the physician has excised the cyst, the circulator will hold the formalin bottle to catch the specimen. The formalin bottle is not sterile. Circulator will cover with lid immediately. The bottle should already be labeled appropriately for transport to the laboratory.		
12. Assist the physician with the suturing by cutting the sutures and blotting.		
13. On completion, cover tray so the patient does not see. Take care of the patient. *Patients have a tendency for syncope after procedures. Sharps and other bodily fluids are best covered both preop and postop.*		
14. Remove gloves and wash hands. Demonstrate postop care and answer any questions the patient may have. Thank the patient and escort to the reception or recovery area.		
15. Return to the room and tear down the tray and clean room according to OSHA standards.		
16. Ready the specimen and laboratory requisition for transportation to the laboratory. A call to the carrier will signify a pick up. Role-play.		
17. Using the techniques taught, prepare instruments for wrapping and autoclaving.		
18. Wash hands. Document.		

Key: Satisfactory = S; Unsatisfactory = U

Preop/Postop Instructions

Preop: Arrive 15 minutes early. Purchase triple antibiotic ointment, hydrogen peroxide, and sterile 4x4 gauze bandages or ready-made sterile bandages before the surgery. Call ahead if there is any change in your health status.

Postop: Taking care of the surgical site is just as important as what the physician just did. Several times a day, remove old dressing and clean incision with a 50% mixture of warm water and hydrogen peroxide. Do not saturate the site. The sutures are not to get wet for 7 days. When showering/bathing, cover area with clean wrap. Keep the site free of crusting and scabbing. A small amount of oozing is normal. Anything more should be reported to the physician. Apply a generous amount of antibiotic ointment, and cover with new sterile bandage/gauze. The physician has prescribed penicillin 500 mg. You are to take two pills two times a day. You must finish the entire prescription for the medication to work. The antibiotic will help keep infection away. The physician will see you in F/U in 5–7 days to remove the sutures.

Remember: You document only your part in the surgery because the physician will dictate or chart the Op Report. You are responsible for the preop and postop, patient home care instructions, and follow-up visits.

PROGRESS NOTE – DOCUMENTATION

Name Student/Patient _____

DOB _____

Allergies _____

Preop Vitals

Date _____

_____

_____

T _____   BP _____   P _____   R _____

_____

_____

Lab/Pathology sent to _____

Instructor Comments _____

_____

_____

Practicum 29. Assisting With Oral Medications

COMPETENCY

CAAHEP: 3. b. (4) (g) Apply pharmacology principles to prepare and administer **oral** and parenteral
(excluding IV) medications

ABHES: 4. (m) Prepare and administer medications as directed by physicians

SPECIFIC TASK

The physician (instructor) will give you a verbal /written order to administer an **ORAL** medication to the patient in the office. You will need to adhere to all Guidelines to Administering Medication, OSHA Guidelines, and PPE.

You will calculate, prepare, and administer the medication in the time specified by your instructor. The student will document the actual order regardless of what is used as the medication. Your instructor may choose a liquid or pill form or both.

Suggestions: Role-play using a classmate as the patient. Either use a piece of candy/soda as the oral medication or use a real/mock medication and the classmate will just pretend to swallow.

STANDARD PRECAUTIONS

OSHA regulations, PPE, sharps, biohazard container, soap, and water

EQUIPMENT/SUPPLIES

Oral medication, medication cup, patient chart/progress note, Physician's Desk Reference (PDR), medication tray, cup for water if necessary, knowledge of medication and any side effects

STANDARD OF PERFORMANCE OF THE TASK

You may earn a maximum of 5 points for each competency regardless of the number of steps to be performed.

EX: If you miss two steps and achieve all the rest then you have earned 3 points.

More than five steps missed means that you have 0 points.

Your instructor may choose not to assign points but check you off on a pass or fail status. Regardless, you may need to repeat the competency for successful completion.

It is up to your instructor to determine the maximum number of tries before the competency has been met successfully in the time allotted.

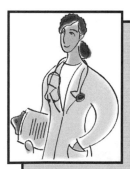

Make a Difference

The Seven Rights of Drug administration is one of the most important aspects when administering medication. Always remember these rights when you become a practitioner and you will keep yourself and the patient free of liabilities associated with medical errors. Remember that the dose you have on hand is not always the dose you want. You may have to perform dosage calculations to obtain the amount ordered by the physician. Always double-check your work for accuracy and ask if you don't know!

Student Name: _____ Date: _____

Time: Satisfactory   Unsatisfactory

Successful Completion: Yes   No

Grade/Points: _____   Pass   Fail

Need to Repeat: _____   Number of Attempts: 1   2   3

Instructor Comments: _____

_____

_____

Patient Name: Ethel Burke
Current Meds: Digoxin 0.125 mg – 1/day; Estrace 1 mg – 1/day; Allegra 60 mg – 1/day; Glucotrol 5 mg – 1/day. No difficulty swallowing any type of oral medication. The patient does wear dentures.
Allergies: Penicillin

Verbal/Written Order _____

(The instructor will provide you with the order here)

CONDITIONS UNDER WHICH THE STUDENT IS EXPECTED TO PERFORM THE TASK

Follow Task/Performance Steps

Task/Performance Step	S	U
1. Verify the written/verbal order to administer an oral medication **Right Route.**		
2. If you are not familiar with the drug, look it up in the PDR before assessing the patient. *If the patient has questions about the drug, you will be prepared to answer them. It is also wise to know the drug for case management purposes. Verify the drug ordered is not contraindicated with anything else the patient might be taking.*		
3. Knock on examination room door. Greet patient, identify yourself and confirm you have the **Right Patient.**		
4. Assess the patient history: **Right Time.** Are there allergies to any medications? Have they had this medication before and if so how did they tolerate it? Can the patient tolerate an oral medication by swallowing without difficulty? *Not all patients can take oral medications and it may need to be given in another form.*		
5. Instruct the patient that if it is the first time taking the medication, you will have them wait in the office for observation. *Reminder: Especially medication such as penicillin. Many people develop allergies later in life. It is safer to have the patient wait so you can react to any adverse reactions.*		
6. Ask the patient if there are any questions and answer. Let the patient know you will go and prepare the medication and return.		

7.	Verifying the order again, find the appropriate medication. Check the label and make sure it is the correct medication ordered. **Right Drug.** *Reminder: Some dosages may not be what the physician ordered, so you would need to calculate based on dose you have to dose you want. All medications will vary. Remember, if you are ever unsure, ask someone to verify or assist you.*		
8.	Wash hands and gather the rest of the supplies. Work in a well-lighted area where there are no distractions.		
9.	Check the drug expiration date, name, strength, and appearance of the product. Calculate the appropriate dosage. **First Time.**		
10.	For tablets, capsules, spanules, etc., pour the desired number of pills into the medicine cup without touching the lid to the cup. This can be done by pouring the pills into the cap then into the cup. This prevents waste or contamination. *Reminder: Never pour back into the bottle any pills that have spilled. The containers are usually sterile inside. Never give oral medication from your hand or directly from the tray. Oral medication should always be in a medicine cup. For liquid medication the same applies, never touch the rim of the bottle to anything. Hold the bottle at eye level with the label away from the side you are pouring from.* *Reminder: Never administer or give a patient medication where the label is soiled and it is not legible. Discard the medication in the appropriate container or according to your office protocol. Do not guess even if you know that it is the correct medication. Liability is a concern, so by sticking to all the cardinal rules you can never go wrong.*		
11.	While replacing the cap, check the medication for the **Second Time**. Return to the storage area and check the label for the **Third Time**.		
12.	Assemble your tray with a cup of water if appropriate and the medication cup with the medication in it. *Reminder: Most liquid medication will not require that a drink be taken at the same time. Consult your PDR if you are not familiar with the medication.*		
13.	Carrying the medication tray, knock on door, and identify yourself to the patient.		
14.	Explain the medication and how to take it (pills verses liquid). Hand the medicine cup to the patient so you do not touch the medication. **Right Technique**. Explain again that you will have the patient wait if necessary for observations. Discard items from tray in appropriate containers and wash hands.		
15.	Check on patient status. Thank the patient and escort to the reception area with any further instructions.		
16.	Document. **Right Documentation.**		

Key: Satisfactory = S; Unsatisfactory = U

PROGRESS NOTE – DOCUMENTATION

Name Student/Patient _____

DOB _____

Allergies _____

Date _____

_____

_____

_____

_____

_____

_____

Instructor Corrections _____

_____

_____

_____

_____

_____

Practicum 30. Assisting With Parenteral Medications

COMPETENCY

CAAHEP: 3. b. (4) (g) Apply pharmacology principles to prepare and administer oral and **parenteral** (excluding IV) medications

ABHES: 4. (m) Prepare and administer medications as directed by physicians

SPECIFIC TASK

Correctly calculate and withdraw medication, checking the label three times and administer an **Intradermal, Subcutaneous,** and/or **Intramuscular** injection after receiving a written/verbal order by a physician/instructor.

Be sure to use correct needle/syringe sizes, follow the Seven Guidelines to Administering Medication, and use proper OSHA and PPE within the time allotted by the instructor.

Your instructor may choose to provide an order for all three and/or a combination of routes to satisfy this competency.

STANDARD PRECAUTIONS

Hand washing, gloves/PPE, sharps, biohazard container, antiseptic

EQUIPMENT/SUPPLIES

Medication order/medication tray
Patient chart/progress note
Vial/ampule of medication (MDV 0.9% sodium chloride for injecting, optional)
Correct sterile needle/syringe unit
Antiseptic wipe for patient and medication vial/cotton ball
Disposable gloves
Sharps container (no recapping of needles)
PDR (to look up unfamiliar medication)
Band-Aid if applicable

STANDARD OF PERFORMANCE OF THE TASK

You may earn a maximum of 5 points for each competency regardless of the number of steps to be performed.

EX: If you miss two steps and achieve all the rest then you have earned 3 points.

More than five steps missed means that you have 0 points.

Your instructor may choose not to assign points but check you off on a pass or fail status.

Regardless, you may need to repeat the competency for successful completion.

It is up to your instructor to determine the maximum number of tries before the competency has been met successfully in the time allotted.

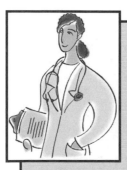

Make a Difference

Administering medication is a serious responsibility. Adhering to the standards will keep you and the patient out of harm's way. Always follow and adhere to FDA and DEA regulations and suggested guidelines. Know what kind of medication you are dealing with before you administer it to your patient.

Student Name: _____   Date: _____

Time: Satisfactory   Unsatisfactory

Successful Completion: Yes   No

Grade/Points: _____   Pass   Fail

Need to Repeat: _____   Number of Attempts: 1   2   3

Instructor Comments: _____

_____

_____

Patient Name: Phyllis IsGood
Allergies: Biaxin and Imitrex
Fractured left arm
Tolerates injections well

Verbal/Written Order _____
                              (The instructor will provide you with the order here.)

CONDITIONS UNDER WHICH THE STUDENT IS EXPECTED TO PERFORM THE TASK

Follow Task/Performance Steps

Task/Performance Step	S	U
1. Perform medical asepsis hand wash. Adhere to OSHA guidelines.		
2. Verify the written/verbal order. Check insert or PDR for drug unfamiliarity with contraindications or side effects.		
3. Greet patient, identify yourself, identify the patient. **Right Patient**.		
4. Ask pertinent questions: Allergies to medication; has patient ever had this medication before; how does patient tolerate injections.		
5. Patient education: May be necessary to wait in office 15–30 minutes if first time for medication; contraindications and/or possible side effects; RTC if the injection test results need to be read in your office.		
6. Again, compare the order with the medication and the patient to ensure the correct name of the patient and the right time to administer the drug. **Right Time.**		
7. Assess the patient for size of needle, site, and explain the procedure. **Right Route.**		
8. Don nonsterile gloves.		
9. Prepare the equipment needed, working in a well-lighted, quiet, clean area. Check syringes and needles for sterility or defects. Needle and syringe packages should not have seal broken.		
10. Locate the correct medication, **Right Drug,** from the storage area or refrigerator and check against your order. (Roll refrigerated medications gently between palms of hands to warm.)		
11. Check for drug expiration date, name, **First Time,** strength, and appearance of the product.		
12. Calculate appropriate dosage. Attach needle or check unit for tightness on syringe if unit comes as one. Prepare the syringe, pull back stopper to loosen, pull stopper back (ordered amount of medication) to fill syringe with air.		

13. With antiseptic wipe, cleanse the top of rubber stopper of the medication vial. Discard wipe.		
14. Check medication label. **Second Time.** Invert medication gently if required for mixing. With syringe in one hand and vial in other, holding vial vertically, upside down at eye level with label away from you, inject air from syringe into medication vial.		
15. Withdraw desired amount of medication into the syringe. **Right Dose.** Tap lightly to rid syringe of air bubbles. Invert vial and syringe and withdraw needle.		
16. With needle guard on medication tray, gently slide needle into guard.		
17. Check medication for the **Third Time** and replace to storage area. If giving an IM injection it may be necessary to switch to a new needle. It is common to draw with one needle and inject with another. The needle you drew with is now contaminated and dulled.		
18. Take medication tray to patient. Position patient for comfort and to reduce strain. Expose site.		
19. Cleanse site with antiseptic wipe using a circular motion starting center of site and moving outward from the center.		
20. Remove sheath from needle. • **ID:** Pull skin taut with thumb of one hand to help give you resistance and hold the syringe with thumb and four fingers in the other hand. Holding the syringe at a 15-degree angle, tell the patient there will be a "little stick," and insert needle through the skin about 1/8 inches. The needle should be transparent through the skin. **Right Technique.** • Do not aspirate. Rotate bevel downward by turning the syringe to 180 degrees to help prevent medication from breaking the skin. • Steadily and not too fast, inject the medication, creating a wheal. • Do not massage. Lightly blot dry with a cotton swab. Do not cover with Band-Aid.		
21. Remove sheath from needle. • **SC:** Pull skin taut with thumb of one hand to help give you resistance and hold the syringe with thumb and four fingers in the other hand. Holding the syringe at a 45-degree angle, tell the patient there will be a "little stick," and insert needle quickly at designated site. • Release skin, switch hands to ensure steadiness, keeping your eye on the site and aspirate. Withdraw immediately if any blood is seen in syringe and repeat entire procedure using another site, new medication, and syringe unit. **Right Technique.** • Administer the medication at a consistent rate. A rapid injection could cause tissue trauma. • With dry cotton swab in one hand, withdraw syringe holding cotton on site while applying pressure to the site injected. Gently massage unless contraindicated. Apply bandage to site over cotton for pressure and prevention of contamination to the site.		

22. Remove sheath from needle. • **IM:** With thumb and first two fingers grasp site muscle and pull away from the bone. Holding the syringe like a dart at a 90-degree angle, tell the patient there will be a "little stick," and insert needle quickly at designated site. Release muscle, switch hands to ensure steadiness, keeping your eye on the site, and aspirate. Withdraw immediately if any blood is seen in syringe and repeat entire procedure using another site, new medication, and syringe unit. **Right Technique.** • Administer the medication at a consistent rate. A rapid injection could cause muscle trauma. • With dry cotton swab in one hand, withdraw syringe holding cotton on site while applying pressure to the site injected. Gently massage unless contraindicated. Apply bandage to site over cotton for pressure and prevention of contamination to the site.		
23. Record the procedure(s) in the patient chart, **Right Documentation,** and on the required DEA form if a Scheduled Drug was used. *A procedure is not complete until documentation has been provided. "If it wasn't documented it wasn't done!"*		

Key: Satisfactory = S; Unsatisfactory = U

PROGRESS NOTE – DOCUMENTATION

Name Student/Patient _____

DOB _____

Allergies _____

Date _____

_____

_____

_____

_____

_____

_____

_____

Instructor Corrections _____

_____

_____

_____

_____

Practicum 31. Medication Records

COMPETENCY

CAAHEP: 3. b. (4) (h) Maintain medication and immunization records
ABHES: 4. (n) Maintain medication records

SPECIFIC TASK

You have received two new patients in your practice, and it is your responsibility to maintain the medication and immunization records of each patient. Each patient has provided you with a list of medication and the most current immunizations. In the time specified by your instructor, complete the attached records by transferring the patient data into the patient medication/immunization record.

PATIENT #1

Larry Droflit: Age – 46 y, DOB: 4/23/58, Male

Adult – Patient #1 List – Medications

Medication Name	Prescription Date	Ordering physician
Tagamet 1 Tab 400 mg hs po	Rx – 4-21-02	Dr. Razul Smit
Calan 1 Cap 80 mg bid po	Rx – 5-25-03	Dr. Shana Organoe
Lasix 1 Tab 20 mg bid po	Rx – 4-21-04	Dr. Razul Smit
Slow K 1 Tab 600 mg qd po	Rx – 5-25-04	Dr. Shana Organoe
Phenergan Suppository 50 mg q4h PRN prn nausea	Rx – 6-23-04	Dr. Franklin Pierce Wright

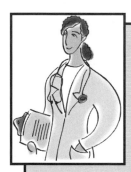

Make a Difference

Many times patients will see more than one's physician. The task of keeping track of one's medication is not easy, but it is important. Too often there are contraindications that would prohibit a patient from being on certain types of medication; therefore, a medication record is kept. Always ask patients what medications they are currently taking or have there been any new meds prescribed since they were last seen. Childhood immunizations protect us from disease, viruses, and bacteria. Maintaining immunization records are important because of the different schedules associated with administering these immunizations. This applies to both adult and pediatric administration. Childhood immunizations should be given at regular intervals, or they are not effective. Can you imagine a world without this type of protection?

PATIENT #2

Phyllis Droflit: Age – 18 mo, DOB 10/14/04, Female

Pediatric – Patient #2 List – Immunizations

Vaccine	Date Given
Hep B 1	January 12, 2004
IPV/OPV 1	January 12, 2004 (IPV 2 and 4 mo given)
MMR 1	February 18, 2004
DPaT 1	February 18, 2004
DPaT 2	May 16, 2005
Hib 1	January 12, 2005

(No reactions noted)
(Administered by Tami Etagnut, MD [Pediatrician])

STANDARD PRECAUTIONS

NA

EQUIPMENT/SUPPLIES

Black and red pen
Medication/immunization record
Patient record/chart.

STANDARD OF PERFORMANCE OF THE TASK

You may earn a maximum of 5 points for each competency regardless of the number of steps to be performed.

> EX: If you miss two steps and achieve all the rest then you have earned 3 points.

> More than five steps missed means that you have 0 points.

> Your instructor may choose not to assign points but check you off on a pass or fail status.

Regardless, you may need to repeat the competency for successful completion.

> It is up to your instructor to determine the maximum number of tries before the competency has been met successfully in the time allotted.

Student Name: _____ Date: _____

Time: Satisfactory   Unsatisfactory

Successful Completion: Yes   No

Grade/Points: _____   Pass   Fail

Need to Repeat: _____ Number of Attempts: 1   2   3

Instructor Comments: _____

_____

_____

CONDITIONS UNDER WHICH THE STUDENT IS EXPECTED TO PERFORM THE TASK

Follow Task/Performance Steps

	Task/Performance Step	S	U
1.	Wash hands. Obtain the patient record.		
2.	Knock on door. Greet patients, identify yourself, and confirm the patient names.		
3.	Explain that the physician would like to start a record of the prior medical history for medication and immunizations and that you would like to review the list the patient has brought with them. There may be some questions if you do not understand the list. *Reminder: For the pediatric patient, remember to gain trust and confidence. Eye level with children works well. (With this scenario the child is too young to communicate, but always work on trust and confidence right from the beginning).*		
4.	Obtain list from parent and thoroughly review. Ask any questions that are pertinent to the record. Document the new list of medications and immunizations on the medications records included in this competency.		
5.	Once completed, read what you have written back to the parent/patient and confirm that you have the correct information.		
6.	Ask if there are any questions that you can answer. Thank the patients and escort them to the reception area.		
7.	Prepare the examination room for the next patient. Wash hands.		

Key: Satisfactory = S; Unsatisfactory = U

SMART THINKING

Learning about immunizations will help you understand how you can deliver better patient education. Look in your textbook, PDR, or reference library and provide the description of each immunization listed below. Remember, practice makes perfect.

Disease	Immunization	Description
Diphtheria	DTaP, Td	
Pertussis		
Tetanus		
Hepatitis B	Hep B	

Disease	Immunization	Description
Measles, Mumps, Rubella (German measles)	MMR	
Haemophilus influenzae or meningitis	Hib	
Pneumococcal disease	PCV-7	
Polio	OPV	
Varicella zoster (Chicken pox)	Var	

PATIENT MEDICATION RECORD

Patient's Name _____

DOB _____

Sex _____

Orig. Rx Order Date	Today's Date	Dosage	Route	Patient Concerns	Ordering Physician	Current Use	Initials

IMMUNIZATION RECORD

Patient's Name _____

DOB _____

Sex _____

Vaccine*	Date Given	Physician Name/ Local HD Stamp	Next Dose Due	Reaction	Initials
DTAP					
1					
2					
3					
4					
Age 4–6 mo					
IPV					
2 mo					
4 mo					
OPV					
12–18 mo					
4–6 mo					
HIB					
1					
2					
3					
4					
HEP B					
1					
2					
3					
MMR					
12–15 mo					
OTHER					

*Always chart the lot or manufacturer number of each immunization in patient record.

Practicum 32. Risk Management

COMPETENCY

CAAHEP: 3. b. (4) (i) Screen and follow up test results
ABHES: 4. (l) Screen and follow up patient test results
5. (h) Perform risk-management procedures

SPECIFIC TASK

Using the attached laboratory result for the patient Jasan Fordlit, screen results for any abnormal value. Perform risk management by highlighting the abnormal results for the physician.

Show results to the physician (instructor). After the physician has reviewed the results and upon instructions from the physician, role-play with a classmate and call the patient for further testing or give the patient the instructions that the physician requests. Document the results and the conversation with the patient. Screening should take less than 10 minutes to perform.

Patient: Jason Fordlit

DOB: 8/26/84

Previous Lab Results: December 18, 2004

Patient: Jason Fordlit   **DOB**: August 26, 1984
Test: Complete Blood Count (CBC)

Test	Normal Value	Patient Value
RBC	Male: 4.5–6.2 mm; Female: 4–5.5 mm	5.8
WBC	4500–11,000	9450
Hemoglobin	Male: 14–18 g/dL; Female: 12–16 g/dL	14
Hematocrit	Male: 40%–54%; Female: 37%–47%	46%
Platelet	150,000–400,000	200,000

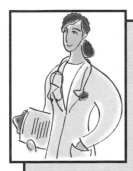

Make a Difference

When screening test results, it is always better to double-check what you are looking at several times. Distractions can cause errors. The patient will incur a negative impact if results are screened or read incorrectly. Good risk-management practices are informing patients of test results, making sure results are documented, and showing that the diagnostic tests are received and reviewed by the physician in a timely manner. Always have the physician initial any patient results and get clarification as to how the physician would like you to proceed.

STANDARD PRECAUTIONS

PPE, soap, and water

EQUIPMENT/SUPPLIES

Attached laboratory results
Patient record/attached progress note
Black pen
Phone

STANDARD OF PERFORMANCE OF THE TASK

You may earn a maximum of 5 points for each competency regardless of the number of steps to be performed.

EX: If you miss two steps and achieve all the rest then you have earned 3 points.

More than five steps missed means that you have 0 points.

Your instructor may choose not to assign points but check you off on a pass or fail status.

Regardless, you may need to repeat the competency for successful completion.

It is up to your instructor to determine the maximum number of tries before the competency has been met successfully in the time allotted.

Student Name: _____   Date: _____

Time:	Satisfactory	Unsatisfactory
Successful Completion:	Yes	No
Grade/Points: _____	Pass	Fail
Need to Repeat: _____	Number of Attempts: 1 2 3	

Instructor Comments: _____

_____

_____

CONDITIONS UNDER WHICH THE STUDENT IS EXPECTED TO PERFORM THE TASK

Follow Task/Performance Steps

	Task/Performance Step	S	U
1.	Student gathers supplies, obtains patient laboratory results, and confirms laboratory results to correct patient medical record by confirming DOB or other identifying information. *Always compare patient name on laboratory results to patient medical record to ensure correct results with correct patient.*		
2.	Student reviews laboratory results and highlights any value that does not fall within the noted normal value range. *Student must be able to recognize abnormal and "panic" value laboratory results to bring to the physician's attention.*		
3.	Student compares current laboratory results to previous laboratory results. If there are significant changes to the current laboratory results, the student highlights previous results. *Comparing previous laboratory values with current laboratory values can be an indicator as to the effectiveness of patient treatment or an improvement or worsening of a patient's condition.*		
4.	Student follows office protocol by bringing directly to physician's (instructors) attention.		
5.	Student ensures that the physician initials the laboratory result after reviewing, which ensures proper risk management control. *For liability issues and to ensure patient results are not overlooked, student should always be sure physician has initialed any laboratory result reviewed and document in patient record. Never file any patient result that has not yet been reviewed.*		
6.	Following physician (instructor) instructions, student notes treatment or next step to be taken regarding abnormal laboratory values.		
7.	Student follows physician order and notifies patient by phone.		
8.	Using proper telephone technique, student notifies patient of current laboratory values and physician request for follow-up lab (CBC) in 1 week. *Be sure you have identified that you are speaking with the patient, and do not give out any patient information to anyone other than the patient.*		

9.	Student schedules patient for follow-up laboratory test and gives any appropriate instructions relative to laboratory test to be drawn. *Special instructions may include fasting before a laboratory draw or instructions to a laboratory facility if lab is not drawn in your office.*		
10.	Student verifies patient understands with patient verbal feedback. *Verifying information with patient ensures patient understands and decreases possible miscommunication.*		
11.	Student communicates to patient that the patient will be notified and scheduled for a follow-up appointment once the new laboratory results have come back. *Patient needs to know what the next plan of action will be once the lab has been drawn.*		
12.	Student documents all interaction with the physician and with the patient in the patient medical record.		

Key: Satisfactory = S; Unsatisfactory = U

PROGRESS NOTE – DOCUMENTATION

Name Student/Patient _____

DOB _____

Allergies _____

Date _____

_____

_____

_____

_____

Instructor Corrections _____

_____

_____

_____

Patient: Jason Fordlit   **DOB**: August 26, 1984
Test: Complete Blood Count (CBC)

Test	Normal Value	Patient Value
RBC	Male: 4.5–6.2 mm; Female: 4–5.5 mm	4.8
WBC	4500–11,000	13,450
Hemoglobin	Male: 14–18 g/dL; Female: 12–16 g/dL	16
Hematocrit	Male: 40%–54%; Female: 37%–47%	48%
Platelet	150,000–400,000	160,000

Practicum 33. Venipuncture/Standard Precaution

COMPETENCY

CAAHEP: 3. b. (1) (d) Dispose of biohazardous materials
3. b. (1) (e) Practice standard precaution
3. b. (2) (a) Perform venipuncture
3. c. (2) (e) Document appropriately

ABHES: 4. (q) Dispose of biohazardous materials
4. (r) Practice standard precaution
4. (s) Perform venipuncture
5. (b) Document accurately

SPECIFIC TASK

Perform venipuncture using the evacuated tube system in the correct order of draw as though you were sending the tests to a laboratory for evaluation and interpretation of the tests. Document the procedure. Standard precautions and proper disposal of biohazard materials must be adhered to as well as the proper use of waste receptacles.

VERBAL/WRITTEN ORDER

CBC with differential
Protime
Digoxin level

STANDARD PRECAUTIONS

Gloves, protective eye shield, laboratory coat, soap and warm water, sharps containers, biohazard waste receptacles

EQUIPMENT/SUPPLIES

Evacuated tube supplies (needles, needle adaptor, collection tubes), antiseptic, cotton or sterile gauze squares, tourniquet, tube rack, sterile bandage or tape, appropriate chair or examination table, laboratory requisition form, biohazard plastic bag for transportation of specimen, ammonia inhalant, PPE, and biohazard waste containers

STANDARD OF PERFORMANCE OF THE TASK

You may earn a maximum of 5 points for each competency regardless of the number of steps to be performed.
EX: If you miss two steps and achieve all the rest then you have earned 3 points.
More than five steps missed means that you have 0 points.
Your instructor may choose not to assign points but check you off on a pass or fail status.
Regardless, you may need to repeat the competency for successful completion.
It is up to your instructor to determine the maximum number of tries before the competency has been met successfully in the time allotted.

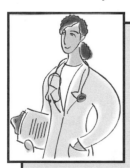

Make a Difference

Practicing standard precaution, proper use of biohazard containers, and barrier protection will keep you safe and create a safe work environment. When working with sharps, safety should be your number one concern.

Student Name: _____   Date: _____

Time: Satisfactory   Unsatisfactory

Successful Completion: Yes   No

Grade/Points: _____   Pass   Fail

Need to Repeat: _____   Number of Attempts: 1   2   3

Instructor Comments: _____

_____

_____

CONDITIONS UNDER WHICH THE STUDENT IS EXPECTED TO PERFORM THE TASK

Follow Task/Performance Steps

Task/Performance Step	S	U
1. Confirm the verbal/written order for the test to be performed. Perform a medical aseptic hand wash.		
2. Gather all the necessary supplies into the area where the venipuncture will be performed.		
3. Assemble the equipment so you are not doing it in front of the patient. Have your bandage, antiseptic, and gauze/cotton ready. *Seeing needles before the procedure can bring alarm to pediatric patients as well as adult and geriatric patients. Being prepared displays professionalism and good time management.*		
4. Prepare the needle adaptor by inserting the threaded luer-lock side of the needle into the adaptor. Twist in a clockwise motion.		
5. Label the collection tubes with the patient name, the name of the test being performed, the physician's name, and the date.		
6. Completely fill out the laboratory requisition form, which will be sent to the laboratory along with the specimen(s).		
7. Greet the patient and introduce yourself. Identify the patient. (If the patient has a common name, ask another identifying question, such as DOB.) (In hospital, identify by comparing the name on the laboratory order to the identification bracelet the patient is wearing.) *For pediatric or elderly patients, ask the parent or guardian or the person who has accompanied them to the appointment.*		
8. Explain the procedure and the purpose of it. Confirm that the patient has followed any instructions before having the test performed for quality assurance of the test, e.g., Was the patient NPO 12 hours as instructed.		
9. Ask the patient if he/she has a preference of which arm is used. Most patients who have had this procedure before know where their best veins are.		

10. Ask the patient if they have ever had this procedure before and if so how did they tolerate it. *There are patients who faint (syncope) during venipuncture technique. If the patient states they do not do well, then lay the patient down from the start and have your ammonia inhalant available. It may be necessary to use a form of restraint, have the parent assist, or both or have the parent wait outside the room until the procedure has been performed on a pediatric patient who will not cooperate during the procedure.*		
11. Wash your hands using friction to generate enough lather for thorough cleansing. Adequately wash between fingers and on wrists, rinsing hands in a downward position. Dry hands with clean paper towel and use paper towel to turn off faucet if it is not automatic. Discard paper towel in proper container. Don clean disposable examination gloves.		
12. If the patient has not given a preference for which arm, assess both arms and sites for the best puncture site.		
13. Apply the tourniquet to the patient's forearm about 2–3 in from the antecubital site. *To apply a proper tourniquet, use both hands and stretch the material on both sides, crossing and meeting with an "x" in the center and top. Grasp this "x" with your first finger and thumb. Next, with your right hand, take the strip of material that overlaps the top and to your right where the "x" is and snugly slip it in under your "x" creating a loop. If you were left-handed it would be the opposite.*		
14. Ask the patient to open and close their fist until you tell them to stop. Find a vein by palpating the site using your index finger. *Opening and closing the fist will help build pressure so the blood will flow easily. Tourniquets should not be left on for more than 1 minute at a time. This can prevent the flow of blood and cause the blood to hemolyze prematurely. If a site cannot be determined, release the tourniquet, wait 1–2 minutes and try again. Ask the patient to stop making a fist.*		
15. After a site as been determined, remove the tourniquet and cleanse the site with antiseptic wipe, gauze, or cotton and 70% alcohol. Start in the middle of the site using a circular motion and continue the circular motion wiping the germs outward away from the center of the site to be punctured. Do not wipe over the same spot more than once.		
16. Allow the site to air dry. *Blowing or wiping will recontaminate the site and could cause possible infection to the site.*		
17. Reapply the tourniquet to the patient's arm. Ask him/her to open and close a fist until you tell say stop.		
18. Remove the plastic cap from your needle and quickly check the needle for any defects or spurs. To hold the patient's skin taut and to keep the veins from rolling, anchor the skin just below the insertion site with your thumb.		
19. At a 15-degree angle, bevel side of needle up, aligned parallel to the vein, quickly and smoothly insert the needle to a depth of 0.25 to 0.5 in. *You can sometimes go beyond the vein, hit the vein wall, or not go in far enough. Proper technique of insertion is important for a quality assurance specimen. Some patients will require a different depth of insertion depending on how deep or how superficial their veins are.*		
20. Lift your anchoring thumb and grasp the needle adaptor with your thumb and forefinger to help secure that the needle will not move. With the other hand, firmly seat the collection tube into place over the needlepoint, puncturing the rubber stopper allowing the blood to flow. Collect the correct amount of blood for the specimen you are obtaining and withdraw the tube.		

21. Invert tube gently if there is additive and place in the tube rack upright. If there is no additive, simply place in the tube rack upright. *Blood coagulates very fast, so tubes should not be placed on their side because this compromises the quality of the specimen.*		
22. Switch tubes by pulling the existing tube out and inserting the next using a steady and smooth motion. Keep your eye on the needle at all times so as not to compromise your draw or the patient site.		
23. Once the blood is flowing freely, you may ask your patient to release their fist.		
24. When the last tube is almost full, remove the tourniquet by pulling the end of the tucked-in loop. *Tourniquets tied too tight may cut off blood flow. Tourniquets that are removed too quickly before all the specimens are obtained can result in slow flow or none at all. Always try to adhere to the 1-minute rule. **Always:** tourniquets should be removed before the tube is removed or the needle is withdrawn.*		
25. Withdraw the needle quickly and smoothly by placing a cotton or sterile gauze on the site over the needle and pulling the needle out. If you are using a safety device, activate it at this time. Do not recap needles. Do not lay the needle down on any surface. Dispose of the needle immediately in the proper sharps container.		
26. Continue to hold pressure for 1–2 minutes on the site while applying the bandage or tape. It is a good idea to leave the gauze or cotton under the applied bandage for extra pressure.		
27. Instruct the patient about care of the puncture site at this time and encourage questions. Do not allow the patient to apply his or her own pressure to the site or get up immediately.		
28. Assess the patient's appearance and the site. Reapply a fresh bandage if necessary. Thank the patient and allow them to leave.		
29. Remove all the material that is considered biohazard waste and place in the biohazard box. This box should be labeled "Biohazard" and contain a red bag for identification purposes.		
30. Sharps are to be carefully handled and disposed of in only containers labeled "Sharps" "Fill 3/4 Full Only." These boxes come in various sizes but should also be red and puncture proof.		
31. Disinfect the work area with disposable paper towels and a disinfectant solution by spraying directly over the area where the specimen was collected or anywhere else that was contaminated during the procedure.		
32. Place tubes in transport bag with laboratory requisition form. Store in appropriate place until pick-up.		
33. Remove your gloves and wash your hands.		
34. Document the procedure.		

Key: Satisfactory = S; Unsatisfactory = U

PROGRESS NOTE – DOCUMENTATION

Name Student/Patient _____

DOB _____

Allergies _____

Date _____

_____

_____

_____

_____

_____

_____

*Always ask the patient if there are any allergies to latex, bandages, or other substances that might touch the patient during the procedure.

EXAMPLE CHARTING

```
VO: CBC with differential (CBC with diff), digoxin level
(dig), protime (PT).

CBC with differential, digoxin level, and protime drawn
from left antecubital area.

Pt. tol. well. Specimens to Bayside Laboratory.

Pt. to RTC in 3 days for results                    KH, CMA
```

Practicum 34. Capillary Puncture

COMPETENCY

CAAHEP: 3. b. (2) (b) Perform capillary puncture
            3. b. (3) (c) CLIA Waived Tests
            (iii) Perform chemistry tests
            3. c. (4) (d) Use methods of quality control

ABHES: 4. (j) Collect and process specimens
            4. (t) Perform capillary puncture
            4. (aa) Perform chemistry testing
            4. (i) Use quality control

SPECIFIC TASK

Perform a real capillary puncture on an adult (classmate) and practice a pediatric capillary puncture on a laboratory doll or foot using the appropriate sites for each. Perform this task according to proper standard and technique.

    Perform a chemistry test by using a CLIA Waived Test and the capillary specimen to determine a blood glucose level. Follow the manufacturer recommendations, steps, and quality control (QC). Document the adult findings and QC within the time specified by your instructor.

VERBAL/WRITTEN ORDER

Capillary puncture for blood glucose level.
Patient: Antonio Cann
DOB: 10/20/27 – No allergies

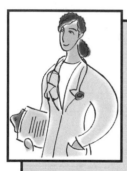

Make a Difference

Sticking the heel of an infant or pediatric patient is never an easy task. The safety of the child should always be the first consideration. Pay close attention to the location and site on the heel as well as the direction of the stick for the adult and pediatric patient. Sticking in any other area of the foot in a child could cause osteomyelitis.

STANDARD PRECAUTIONS

PPE, soap, water, disinfectant

EQUIPMENT/SUPPLIES

Capillary puncture device
Cotton balls
Antiseptic wipes
Sterile adhesive bandage
Blood glucose monitor or CLIA Waived Test kit
Pediatric simulator doll/foot
Normal, low, and high controls
Biohazard containers
Sterile 2x2 gauze
Test strips

STANDARD OF PERFORMANCE OF THE TASK

You may earn a maximum of 5 points for each competency regardless of the number of steps to be performed.

EX: If you miss two steps and achieve all the rest then you have earned 3 points.

More than five steps missed means that you have 0 points.

Your instructor may choose not to assign points but check you off on a pass or fail status.

Regardless, you may need to repeat the competency for successful completion.

It is up to your instructor to determine the maximum number of tries before the competency has been met successfully in the time allotted.

Student Name: _____   Date: _____

Time: Satisfactory   Unsatisfactory

Successful Completion: Yes   No

Grade/Points: _____   Pass   Fail

Need to Repeat: _____   Number of Attempts: 1   2   3

Instructor Comments: _____

_____

_____

CONDITIONS UNDER WHICH THE STUDENT IS EXPECTED TO PERFORM THE TASK

Follow Task/Performance Steps

Task/Performance Step	S	U
1. Student verifies verbal or written physician's order. *Verifying orders beforehand ensures correct laboratory is being collected on correct patient and minimizes incidence of error.*		
2. Student gathers necessary supplies and equipment. Performs aseptic hand wash and puts on personal protective equipment (PPE). *Gathering supplies and equipment ahead of time assists with organization and time management. Hand washing prevents cross-contamination.*		
3. Student greets patient, confirms patient identity, and introduces self.		
4. Student explains procedure and purpose to the patient and confirms patient has followed any special instructions associated with the test being performed. *Example: If test requires fasting, be sure to ask patient the last time they had anything to eat or drink.*		
5. Student asks patient if he/she has had this procedure before and how it was tolerated. *Asking patient before procedure alerts the medical assistant of any potential problems.*		
6. Student assists patient to a sitting or lying-down position. *If your patient does not tolerate this kind of procedure well, lie them down. You may need assistance or restraint for a pediatric patient.*		
7. Student turns on blood glucose monitor, calibrates per manufacturer instructions by matching the code strip number with the appropriate bottle of test strips; tests the normal, high, and low controls; and determines if controls are in acceptable range. **OR** Student follows suggested manufacturer steps for CLIA Waive Test if not using blood glucose machine. Calibrate if necessary and adhere to QC. *Calibrating blood glucose monitor ensures quality control and test reliability.*		
8. Student records test reagent strip control lot number and control results in appropriate place on the attached QC record. **OR** Student follows CLIA kit steps for QC. *Recording reagent strip, lot number, and control results ensures quality control is adhered to and reliability of the test.*		

9. Student examines potential site (fingers for adults, heels for infants) to determine best site to use. *If your patient's site appears cold, warm the site to improve circulation for a successful capillary stick. Warm compresses or commercial heel warmers can be used.*		
10. Student prepares the site with a gentle "milking" or rubbing motion toward the fingertip or heel, keeping the extremity below the heart and cleans area with antiseptic wipe, allowing site to dry. Do not "milk" or massage hard as this can cause bruising and/or can interfere with the specimen results. *"Milking" the site and keeping the site below the heart promotes circulation to the area. Cleaning the area before penetrating the skin removes bacteria from the area and may prevent bacteria from entering the compromised skin.*		
11. For the adult patient, student holds patient's finger between their thumb and forefinger, holding the puncture device at a right angle opposite to the patient's fingerprint.		
12. Student states to patient "there will be a little stick," punctures skin to the side of the pad of the fingertip with a quick, sharp motion, and disposes of the puncture device in appropriate sharps container. *Talking to the patient prepares them for the actual stick and may prevent sudden movement by the patient, which can cause injury.*		
13. For the pediatric/infant, student grasps the heel firmly, holding the puncture device in the opposite hand with the device at an angle opposite the heel print to appropriate area of the heel and punctures with a quick sharp motion. *Heel sticks should only be used on pediatric patients who have not yet started walking. Use appropriate puncture device for pediatric patient to prevent hitting the bone, which can cause osteomyelitis.*		
14. Student allows a drop of blood to form at the puncture site and gently wipes away with sterile 2x2 gauze. *If blood droplet is slow in forming gently "milk" the extremity and avoid pressure to the area, which may hemolyze the specimen. Wiping away the first droplet removes blood that is contaminated with tissue fluid.*		
15. Student follows the CLIA Waived Test instructions for next step or touches the reagent strip to the patient and fills the pad with blood. *If test strip or test pad is not filled or covered completely with blood specimen, this may give inaccurate results.*		
16. After completion of obtaining the specimen, student applies pressure to puncture site with sterile 2x2 gauze or cotton ball until the site has stopped bleeding.		
17. Student waits appropriate time per manufacturer instructions. *Be sure to follow manufacturer instructions due to the many types of blood glucose monitoring systems or CLIA Waived Tests.*		
18. Student observes monitor screen and determines the glucose laboratory value. **OR** Student follows steps in CLIA Waived Test.		
19. Student removes reagent test strip from machine, properly disposes of the strip, and turns off the machine. *Keeping the machine off when not in use will save the life of the battery.*		
20. Student cleans and disinfects work area according to laboratory protocol.		
21. Student removes gloves and washes hands.		
22. Student records glucose result and documents in patient's chart. Student documents QC.		
23. Student checks the puncture site for bleeding and, if necessary, applies adhesive bandage. *For pediatric heel sticks, a bandage is not applied for integrity of the skin and safety of the child.*		

Key: Satisfactory = S; Unsatisfactory = U

QUALITY CONTROL RECORD

Using Glucose Monitor

Dr. Wright says, "Always check chemicals and controls for expiration dates, which will help ensure a more accurate test result."

Date: _____

Normal Control Lot Number: _____

Result: _____

High Control Lot Number: _____

Result: _____

Low Control Lot Number: _____

Result: _____

Patient Result: _____

Blood Glucose Machine Used: _____

Using CLIA Waived Test Kit

QC _____

_____

_____

Patient Result: _____

Test Used: _____

Lot # (if applicable): _____

Patient Documentation: _____

_____

_____

_____

_____

Practicum 35. Microbiology Testing

COMPETENCY

CAAHEP: 3. b. (2) (c) Obtain specimens for microbiological testing
             3. b. (3) (c) CLIA Waived Tests:
             (v) Perform microbiology testing
ABHES: 4. (u) Obtain throat specimen for microbiological testing
             4. (v) Perform wound collection procedure for microbiological testing
             4. (cc) Perform microbiology testing

SPECIFIC TASKS

1. Using a classmate as the patient, role-play and obtain a throat specimen by performing a throat swab from the mucous membranes of the throat. Focus on the tonsil region, the crypts, and the posterior pharynx using a Culturette Collection and Transport System for the purpose of microbiological testing. Document.
2. With a classmate and using a CLIA Waived Strep Test kit; obtain a throat specimen following manufacturer instructions for obtaining the sample, performing the test, and adhering to QC. Document.
3. A classmate will role-play as though there is an infected wound on the left forearm. Perform wound collection by obtaining a specimen from a deep area of the wound. Use the Culturette System. Do not contaminate the wound. Document.

PHYSICIAN'S ORDER

Patient: Jessie Roc
Culture and Sensitivity/Throat. R/O Streptococcus Group A. Send to Bayside Laboratory. Patient to RTC in 3–5 days for results.

Perform Strep Test using CLIA Waived Test in office.

Culture wound on left forearm. Send to Bayside Laboratory for evaluation. R/O Staphylococcus.

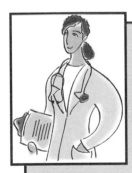

Make a Difference

Adhering to QC will provide you and the patient with accurate results. Always adhere to rules for any time specific tests and check your CLIA Waived Test kit for the expiration date before use.

STANDARD PRECAUTIONS

PPE, soap, water, and disinfectant

EQUIPMENT/SUPPLIES

Light source
Biohazard waste container
Sterile swab or culterette system
CLIA Waived Strep Test
Tongue depressor
Laboratory request slip/transport bag

STANDARD OF PERFORMANCE OF THE TASK

You may earn a maximum of 5 points for each competency regardless of the number of steps to be performed.

EX: If you miss two steps and achieve all the rest then you have earned 3 points.

More than five steps missed means that you have 0 points.

Your instructor may choose not to assign points but check you off on a pass or fail status.

Regardless, you may need to repeat the competency for successful completion.

It is up to your instructor to determine the maximum number of tries before the competency has been met successfully in the time allotted.

Student Name: _____   Date: _____

Time: Satisfactory   Unsatisfactory

Successful Completion: Yes   No

Grade/Points: _____   Pass   Fail

Need to Repeat: _____   Number of Attempts: 1   2   3

Instructor Comments: _____

_____

_____

CONDITIONS UNDER WHICH THE STUDENT IS EXPECTED TO PERFORM THE TASK

Follow Task/Performance Steps

Task/Performance Step	S	U
OBTAIN THROAT SPECIMEN		
1. Student obtains physician order for throat culture and sensitivity. *Verify order from physician to ensure correct test with correct patient. If any questions regarding order, seek clarification from physician.*		
2. Student gathers supplies, performs aseptic hand wash, and applies PPE as indicated.		
3. Student greets patient, confirms patient's identity, and introduces self.		
4. Student discusses purpose of physician order and procedure of test with patient and allows for patient questions with clarification. *Patient should have a clear understanding of procedure and its purpose and be given an opportunity to have questions clarified.*		
5. Student assists patient to sitting position on examination table and ensures light source is directed at the back of the throat. *For pediatric patients, the process may be easier by placing the patient in a supine position. Seek assistance or use a pediatric restraint if necessary.*		
6. Student opens collection system by peeling the paper pack halfway down, removing the swab carefully with dominant hand. *Be sure not to contaminate the sterile swab when removing from package because this could alter the test.*		
7. Student instructs patient to tilt head back and open mouth. *If a pediatric patient refuses to open the mouth and all other attempts to coax patient fail, gently pinch the nostrils closed so the child will open the mouth to breathe.*		
8. Student instructs patient to say "AHHH" and with nondominant hand presses midpoint of the tongue with tongue depressor. *Having patient say "AHHH" raises the uvula out of the way and will decrease the urge to gag. Using the tongue depressor clears the tongue for the specimen path.*		
9. Student carefully directs swab to the back of the throat, swabbing the tonsil region, the crypts, and the posterior pharynx with a twisting motion. *Using a twisting motion enables maximum collection of pathogens. Avoid touching other areas than those of suspected infection.*		

10. Student maintains position of tongue depressor and tongue when withdrawing the swab from the patient's mouth. *Avoiding the tongue while removing the swab prevents contamination of the swab.*		
11. Student removes tongue depressor and disposes in biohazard container.		
12. Student immediately inserts swab back into plastic sleeve and crushes vial of transport medium to moisten the tip of the swab. *Touching the outside of the sleeve could contaminate the specimen. Be sure to always follow manufacturer instructions for transfer of specimen. Improper handling of specimen will alter results.*		
13. Student labels the collection system correctly with patient name, date, time, specimen, and physician name.		
14. Student attaches completed laboratory requisition slip and routes specimen to the laboratory for testing per office protocol. *Be sure to follow office/laboratory protocol regarding storage and transport. Some specimens require refrigeration until the laboratory courier picks them up.*		
15. Student thanks patient and asks if there are any further questions.		
16. Student disinfects area, removes gloves, and disposes appropriately. Washes hands.		
17. Student documents procedure, patient's tolerance, and disposition of specimen in patient's medical record.		
PERFORM CLIA WAIVED STREP TEST		
1. Student obtains verbal/written order.		
2. Follows steps 2–11 in previous competency to obtain specimen or follows manufacturer recommendations from CLIA Waived Strep Test.		
3. Student adheres to quality control/assurance if applicable.		
4. Student performs test according to package instructions.		
5. Student follows steps 15–17 in previous competency.		
6. Documents results and quality control if applicable.		
PERFORMS WOUND COLLECTION		
1. Student obtains verbal or written physician order for wound culture and sensitivity.		
2. Student gathers supplies, performs aseptic hand wash, and applies PPE as indicated.		
3. Student greets patient, confirms patient's identity, and introduces self.		
4. Student discusses purpose of physician order and procedure of test with patient and allows for patient questions with clarification.		
5. Student asks patient if currently taking antibiotics. If so, student documents on laboratory requisition slip. *Labs need to be informed of any patient antibiotic therapy, because antibiotics can hinder bacteria growth when culturing specimen.*		
6. Student assists patient to supine position on examination table.		
7. Student directs light source at wound site for collection. *Good visibility is vital to specimen collection to ensure proper area is cultured and to avoid contamination.*		
8. Student opens collection system by peeling the paper pack halfway down and removing the swab carefully with dominant hand. *Be sure not to contaminate the sterile swab when removing from package, which could alter the test.*		
9. Student examines site. Using nondominant hand holds wound site open gently and carefully, just enough to obtain specimen without further injury to site. *Holding wound open slightly allows for increased visibility and access to inner wound.*		

10. Student carefully directs swab to the deepest area of the wound or area of obvious infectious material and swabs with a twisting motion. *Using a twisting motion enables maximum collection of pathogens. Avoid touching other areas other than those of suspected infection.*		
11. Student immediately inserts swab carefully back into plastic sleeve and crushes vial of transport medium to moisten the tip of the swab.		
12. Student labels the collection system correctly with patient name, date, time, physician name, and wound source. *Be sure to identify wound source (e.g., "Laceration left anterior forearm") on specimen, laboratory requisition, and patient record.*		
13. Student attaches completed laboratory requisition slip and routes specimen to the laboratory for testing per office protocol.		
14. Student thanks patient and asks if there are any further questions.		
15. Student disinfects area, removes gloves, disposes appropriately, and washes hands.		
16. Student documents procedure.		

Key: Satisfactory = S; Unsatisfactory = U

OBTAIN THROAT SPECIMEN – PROGRESS NOTE – DOCUMENTATION

Name Student/Patient _____

Date _____

_____

_____

_____

_____

_____

_____

PERFORM CLIA WAIVED STREP TEST – PROGRESS NOTE – DOCUMENTATION

Name Student/Patient _____

Date _____

_____

_____

_____

_____

_____

_____

PERFORM WOUND COLLECTION – PROGRESS NOTE – DOCUMENTATION

Name Student/Patient _____

Date _____

_____

_____

_____

_____

_____

_____

Instructor Corrections _____

_____

_____

_____

_____

Practicum 36. Urine Collection/Patient Instruction

COMPETENCY

CAAHEP: 3. b. (2) (d) Instruct patients in the collection of a clean-catch mid-stream urine
ABHES: 4. (w) Instruct patient in the collection of a clean-catch mid-stream urine specimen

SPECIFIC TASK

Using a classmate as the patient, instruct and collect a clean-catch mid-stream urine specimen free from contamination using good patient instruction.

STANDARD PRECAUTIONS

PPE, soap, water, disinfectant

EQUIPMENT/SUPPLIES

Sterile urine collection/specimen container or kit
Label/antiseptic wipes/paper towel

STANDARD OF PERFORMANCE OF THE TASK

You may earn a maximum of 5 points for each competency regardless of the number of steps to be performed.
    EX: If you miss two steps and achieve all the rest then you have earned 3 points.
    More than five steps missed means that you have 0 points.
    Your instructor may choose not to assign points but check you off on a pass or fail status.
Regardless, you may need to repeat the competency for successful completion.
    It is up to your instructor to determine the maximum number of tries before the competency has been met successfully in the time allotted.

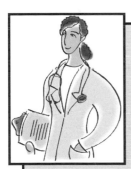

Make a Difference

There is important patient education associated with this task. If the urine becomes contaminated, an accurate result will not be obtained. The tips below will ensure proper collection.

Student Name: _____   Date: _____

Time: Satisfactory   Unsatisfactory

Successful Completion: Yes   No

Grade/Points: _____   Pass   Fail

Need to Repeat: _____   Number of Attempts: 1   2   3

Instructor Comments: _____

_____

_____

CONDITIONS UNDER WHICH THE STUDENT IS EXPECTED TO PERFORM THE TASK

Follow Task/Performance Steps

Task/Performance Step	S	U
1. Student obtains physician/instructor order for mid-stream clean-catch urinalysis.		
2. Student gathers supplies, performs aseptic hand washing.		
3. Student greets patient, confirms patient's identity, and introduces self.		
4. Student discusses purpose of physician order and procedure of test with patient and allows for patient questions with clarification. *Patient should have a clear understanding of procedure and its purpose and be given opportunity to have questions clarified.*		
ASSISTING PATIENT WITH COLLECTION		
5 Student puts on gloves and assists patient to restroom for collection.		
6. Student removes specimen container lid and places lid on clean paper towel with inside facing up. *Laying the lid face down or on unclean surface may contaminate the container and the specimen.*		
7. Student opens the antiseptic wipes containing three wipes and spreads the labia of a female patient with nondominate hand. *Be sure to explain each step of the procedure to the patient as each step is taken as not to cause any undue anxiety for the patient.*		
8. Student takes first wipe to the left labia from top toward the rectum in one swiping motion. Repeats step using second wipe on right labia, and third wipe down the middle. *Cleansing the area before collection ensures QC and less contamination.*		
9. Student maintains spread labia and instructs patient to urinate a small amount into toilet and stop. *Expelling small amounts of urine initially prevents skin surface bacteria from entering the specimen container. It may be difficult for pediatric or geriatric patients to stop voiding, in this case, move the specimen container into the flow of urine until desired amount is obtained.*		
10. Student positions specimen container as close to area as possible and instructs patient to resume urinating until desired amount of urine is obtained. *Be sure not to touch any part of the body, vagina, rectum, or toilet because this will contaminate the specimen.*		

11. Student removes one glove and carefully replaces the lid to the specimen container with the ungloved hand. *Be sure not to touch the inside of the lid, which may contaminate the specimen.*		
12. Student allows patient privacy and offers tissues or towelettes if necessary. Assist patient as needed.		
INSTRUCTION FOR PATIENT COLLECTION		
13. Student instructs patient to perform good hand washing before and after procedure and explains the importance.		
14. Student explains procedure, verifies patient understands procedure, and importance of avoiding contamination.		
15. Student instructs patient on proper collection procedure using steps 6–11. *If patient will be collecting specimen at home be sure patient understands procedure, is given written instruction, and instruct patient to refrigerate urine until brought to office or laboratory.*		
COLLECTING FROM MALE PATIENTS		
16. Student assists or instructs **circumcised** patient to clean head of penis thoroughly with first sterile towelette, clean from the urethral opening in a circular motion outward away from the urethral opening with the second towelette, and repeating with the third towelette. *Cleansing from the urethral opening outward removes bacteria from that source.*		
17. Student instructs or assists patient on proper collection using steps 6–11.		
18. Student instructs or assists **noncircumcised** patient to retract the foreskin with nondominant hand before cleaning following step 16. *Patient may need to be instructed to clean penis after retracting foreskin with soap and water from top downward before preparing for collection. Be sure to have patient rinse well with water as soap can increase pH level.*		
19. Student completes label with patient name, date, and time of collection; physician's name; and initials of person collecting specimen.		
20. Student places specimen and laboratory requisition in biohazard transport bag.		
21. Student disinfects area, removes gloves, and disposes appropriately. Washes hands. *Specimen may need to be stored in refrigerator until transport is possible, be sure to follow office protocol regarding storage and transport.*		
22. Student thanks patient and asks if patient has any further questions and clarifies.		
23. Student documents procedure.		

Key: Satisfactory = S; Unsatisfactory = U

PROGRESS NOTE – DOCUMENTATION

Name Student/Patient _____

Date _____

_____

_____

Instructor Corrections _____

_____

_____

Practicum 37. Hematology Testing

COMPETENCY

CAAHEP: 3. b. (3) (c) CLIA Waived Test
                (ii) Perform hematology testing
ABHES: 4. (z) Perform hematology

SPECIFIC TASK

Using the CLIA Waived Tests below or suggested CLIA approved tests, perform an Erythrocyte Sedimentation Rate (Sed Rate or ESR) using only an EDTA-anticoagulated blood sample for either the Wintrobe ESR or Westergren System using QC within the time allotted for the test. Follow standards and universal precautions.

STANDARD PRECAUTIONS

PPE, soap, water, and disinfectant

EQUIPMENT/SUPPLIES

GENERAL

Paper towels/tissues, Timer–1 hour with alarm, EDTA-anticoagulated whole/venous blood sample, Biohazard container

WINTROBE ERYTHROCYTE SEDIMENTATION RATE

Wintrobe sedimentation tube/rack, Disposable Pasteur pipette

SEDIPLAST DISPOSABLE WESTERGREN ERYTHROCYTE SEDIMENTATION RATE

Sediplast kit, Westergren sedimentation tube, Diluent, Sedivial, and rack

OPTIONS FOR OTHER CLIA APPROVED

Erythrocyte sedimentation rate (nonautomated), Becton Dickinson Sedltainer ESR System

STANDARD OF PERFORMANCE OF THE TASK

You may earn a maximum of 5 points for each competency regardless of the number of steps to be performed.
   EX: If you miss two steps and achieve all the rest then you have earned 3 points.
   More than five steps missed means that you have 0 points.
   Your instructor may choose not to assign points but check you off on a pass or fail status.
Regardless, you may need to repeat the competency for successful completion.
   It is up to your instructor to determine the maximum number of tries before the competency has been met successfully in the time allotted.

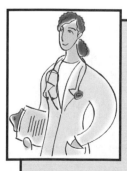

Make a Difference

The ESR is the rate that RBCs fall or settle from the plasma when placed in an upright tube. This is measured by the distance the RBCs travel through the plasma during a given time period. When working with timed tests, make sure you always use a timer and you can hear your alarm/buzzer. Never think that you will just remember because there are too many distractions in this profession.

Student Name: _____   Date: _____

Time: Satisfactory   Unsatisfactory

Successful Completion: Yes   No

Grade/Points: _____   Pass   Fail

Need to Repeat: _____   Number of Attempts: 1   2   3

Instructor Comments: _____

_____

_____

CONDITIONS UNDER WHICH THE STUDENT IS EXPECTED TO PERFORM THE TASK

Follow Task/Performance Steps

Task/Performance Step	S	U
STANDARDS – ALWAYS		
1. Student gathers supplies and equipment. Performs a medical aseptic hand wash and puts on applicable PPE.		
WINTROBE ESR:		
1. Obtains sample.		
2. Mixes the blood sample thoroughly to ensure a well-mixed specimen.		
3. Fills the Pasteur pipette.		
4. Fills the Wintrobe tube to the "0" mark. *Fills from bottom of tube upward to prevent bubble formation.*		
5. Place tube in sedimentation rack in a level position. There should be no extreme temperatures, sunlight, or vibrations and ensure the tube is perfectly vertical. *Inaccurate results may occur if the leveling device is not level.*		
6. Sets time for 1 hour.		
7. After timer sounds at exactly 1 hour, student reads sed rate markings on the tube that measures the distance from the top of the plasma column to the top of the RBCs.		
8. Records results in mL/h.		
9. Discards items and cleans work area using universal precautions.		
SEDIPLAST ERYTHROCYTE SEDIMENTATION RATE		
1. Obtains sample.		
2. Mixes the blood sample thoroughly.		
3. Removes the cap from the Sedivial which should be filled with 3.8% sodium citrate.		
4. With the Pasteur pipette, fills the Sedivial to the indicated line with 0.8 mL of blood.		
5. Mixes the sodium citrate solution and the blood by replacing the stopper in the Sedivial and inverts several times gently.		
6. Student places the sample in the rack in a level position with no vibrations, sunlight, or excessive temperatures.		
7. Using a slight twisting motion, gently insert the sedimentation tube into the Sedivial of blood making sure the tube is inserted all the way. *This will help ensure an accurate reading.*		
8. Sets the timer for 1 hour.		

9. After timer sounds, read the length of the plasma column on the tube.		
10. Records results in mL/h.		
11. Discards items and cleans work area using universal precautions.		

Key: Satisfactory = S; Unsatisfactory = U

PROGRESS NOTE – DOCUMENTATION

Test Used/Identified _____

Results _____

_____

Practicum 38. Immunology Testing

COMPETENCY

CAAHEP: 3. b. (3) (c) CLIA Waived Tests:
(iv) Perform immunology testing
ABHES: 4. (bb) Perform immunology testing

SPECIFIC TASK

Your instructor will choose a CLIA Waived Test for immunology testing. Follow the manufacturer steps using QC and universal precautions in the time specified by your instructor.

SUGGESTED CLIA APPROVED TESTS - IMMUNOLOGY

Helicobacter pylori *Antibodies (for whole blood)*

- Abbott FlexPack HP Test
- Abbott TestPack Plus H. pylori
- Applied Biotech SureStep
- Becton Dickinson LINK 2 H. pylori Rapid Test
- ChemTrak AccuMeter H. pylori Test
- Henry Shein OneStep+ H. pylori Test
- JANT Pharmacal H. pylori Test
- LifeSign Status H. pylori
- Meridian Bioscience Immunocard Stat H. pylori WB Test
- Quidel QuickVue One-Step H. pylori Test
- Quidel QuickVue One-Step H. pylori II Test
- Remel RIM A.R.C. H. pylori Test
- Roche AccuStat H. pylori OneStep
- Trinity Uni-Gold H. pylori

Human Immunodeficiency Virus (HIV) Antibody

- OraSure OraQuick Advance Rapid HIV 1/2 Ab Test (oral fluid, WB fingerstick or venipuncture)
- OraSure Technologies OraQuick Rapid HIV - I Antibody Test
- Trinity Biotech Uni-Gold HIV

Infectious Mononucleosis Antibodies (for whole blood)

- Applied Biotech One Step+ Mono Test
- Applied Biotech SureStep Mono Test
- Applied Biotech Truview Mono Test
- BioStar Acceava Mono Test
- Genzyme Rapid Mono
- Jant Accutest
- LifeSign UniStep Mono
- Polymedco, Inc. Poly stat mono
- Princeton BioMeditech BioSign Mono
- Quidel CARDS O.S. Mono
- Quidel QuickVue+

STANDARD PRECAUTIONS

PPE, soap and water, disinfectant

EQUIPMENT/SUPPLIES

Equipment will vary according to the test you are performing. See your package insert for types of equipment and supplies to have ready.

STANDARD OF PERFORMANCE OF THE TASK

You may earn a maximum of 5 points for each competency regardless of the number of steps to be performed.

    EX: If you miss two steps and achieve all the rest then you have earned 3 points.

    More than five steps missed means that you have 0 points.

    Your instructor may choose not to assign points but check you off on a pass or fail status. Regardless, you may need to repeat the competency for successful completion.

    It is up to your instructor to determine the maximum number of tries before the competency has been met successfully in the time allotted.

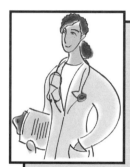

Make a Difference

Immunology is the study of the physical and chemical aspects of one's immunity or resistance to disease or disease process. When a patient's immune system is compromised, the patient is at risk. Always report these kinds of tests to the physician immediately.

Student Name: _____   Date: _____

Time: Satisfactory   Unsatisfactory

Successful Completion: Yes   No

Grade/Points: _____   Pass   Fail

Need to Repeat: _____   Number of Attempts: 1   2   3

Instructor Comments: _____

_____

_____

CONDITIONS UNDER WHICH THE STUDENT IS EXPECTED TO PERFORM THE TASK

Follow Task/Performance Steps

Task/Performance Step	S	U
1. Obtains kit and gathers suggested supplies. Washes hands and puts on appropriate PPE.		
2. Reads test instructions thoroughly asking questions if clarification is needed.		
3. Obtains sample.		
4. Student follows QC and adheres to the steps suggested by the manufacturer.		
5. Washes hands. Student documented any applicable QC and the test result.		
6. Student cleans work area thoroughly using standard precautions. Discards appropriate items in biowaste container.		

Key: Satisfactory = S; Unsatisfactory = U

Test Used/Performed: _____

QC (if applicable): _____

_____

_____

Result: _____

Patient Documentation (if applicable): _____

_____

_____

_____

_____

Practicum 39. Urinalysis/Quality Control

COMPETENCY

CAAHEP: 3. c. (4) (d) Use methods of quality control
                 3. b. (3) (c) CLIA Waived Test
                 (i) Perform urinalysis
ABHES: 4. (i) Use quality control
                 4. (y) Perform urinalysis

SPECIFIC TASK

Collect your own clean-catch urine and perform a chemical analysis of urine using CLIA Waived chemical reagent strips. Your instructor will provide you with strips/bottle/kit. Adhere to and use QC guidelines from the package insert because some of the color strips will require a specific time. Document results and QC.

STANDARD PRECAUTIONS

PPE, soap, water, disinfectant

EQUIPMENT/SUPPLIES

Multistix 10SG or Chemstrip 9
Clock with second hand
Absorbent towel
Urine container/specimen
Color chart (on bottle)
Biohazard container

STANDARD OF PERFORMANCE OF THE TASK

You may earn a maximum of 5 points for each competency regardless of the number of steps to be performed.
    EX: If you miss two steps and achieve all the rest then you have earned 3 points.
    More than five steps missed means that you have 0 points.
    Your instructor may choose not to assign points but check you off on a pass or fail status.
Regardless, you may need to repeat the competency for successful completion.
    It is up to your instructor to determine the maximum number of tries before the competency has been met successfully in the time allotted.

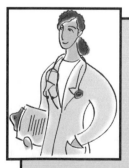

Make a Difference

Color charts with chemical reagent strips will vary depending on the brand. Never memorize the color chart. Always refer to the chart and directions that come with the kit or bottle of strips you are using. Many of the colored strips require more or less time when reading the result. Adhering to time and comparing the patient results to the control strip will ensure QC.

Student Name: _____   Date: _____

Time: Satisfactory   Unsatisfactory

Successful Completion: Yes   No

Grade/Points: _____   Pass   Fail

Need to Repeat: _____   Number of Attempts: 1   2   3

Instructor Comments: _____

_____

_____

CONDITIONS UNDER WHICH THE STUDENT IS EXPECTED TO PERFORM THE TASK

Follow Task/Performance Steps

Task/Performance Step	S	U
1. Student gathers necessary supplies and equipment. Washes hands and puts on PPE. *Urine is considered a bodily fluid. It is best to wear gloves, gown, and a face shield.*		
2. Obtain the urine specimen. *Stale urine is unacceptable for testing for QC of the test. When urine is allowed to stand without refrigeration or without preservatives for more than 1 hour, bacteria can multiply and urine constituents decompose.*		
3. Student checks lot number and expiration date on reagent strip bottle to be used for chemical analysis of urine and records information on the attached Urine Chemistry Quality Control Record. *Expired reagents are not reliable. Recording the lot number and expiration date in the QC record ensures quality control has been adhered to.*		
4. Student removes one reagent strip and recaps container. Reagent strip is dipped into the urine ensuring all pad squares are moist. Tap the strip lightly against the specimen cup to remove excess urine. *Cap should be placed on paper towel or clean surface with inside of cap facing upward to ensure sterility and quality of the reagent bottle. If excessive wetting of the pads occur, the reagents on the pads might be washed away.*		
5. Student holds both the strip and the color chart (found on the bottle) horizontally and lines up the appropriate colors/tests together without touching the bottle to the strip. *Do not touch the test strip to the outside of the bottle upon comparison because this will contaminate the outside of the bottle for future use.*		
6. Checking time intervals per reagent bottle, student compares the color of the reagent pad against the color chart on the bottle and records the results on the urinalysis laboratory form and the Urine Chemistry QC Record using correct units. *Inaccurate reading will occur if the time intervals are not adhered to and will affect the QC of the test. Adequate lighting is essential for accurate color comparison to determine variations in shade.*		
7. Cleans area and discards items appropriately. Washes hands.		

Key: Satisfactory = S; Unsatisfactory = U

URINE CHEMISTRY QC RECORD

Record Control Assayed Values (from package insert).

Patient/Student Name _____ Date _____

Date	Test by	Exp. Date	Cont. Lot Num	pH	Prot.	Gluc	Ket.	Bili	Occ. Bl.	Nitr.	Urob.	Leuk.	Sp. Grav
													1.0___
													1.0___
													1.0___
													1.0___
													1.0___

URINALYSIS

Patient _____ Date _____

TEST	RESULT
Color	
Character	
Glucose	
Bilirubin	
Ketones	
Specific Gravity	
Blood	
Ph	
Protein	
Urobilinogen	
Nitrate	
Leukocytes	
Microscopic Examination	NA
WBC / h.p.f	
RBC / h.p.f	
Casts / l.p.f	
Epithelial Cells	

TEST	RESULT
Bacteria	
Crystals	
Mucous	
Other:	

INSTRUCTOR CORRECTIONS

_____

_____

_____

_____

_____

_____

_____

_____

_____

_____

_____

_____

Practicum 40. Cardiac Testing

COMPETENCY

CAAHEP: 3. b. (3) (a) Perform Electrocardiography
ABHES: 4. (dd) Perform Electrocardiograms
           5. (a) Determine needs for documentation and reporting

SPECIFIC TASK

In the time specified by your instructor, perform a 12-lead electrocardiogram on a classmate who will role-play as the patient. When you escort the patient to the examination room/table, she states she is having chest pain and nausea. You have a standing order to perform an ECG for these situations.

Determine the need for documentation and reporting. Determine the rate and rhythm of the strip and document.

PATIENT INFO

Sara Beaar
Age: 46/Female
DOB: 04/23/68

Medications

Lasix 80 mg 1 qd
Precose 50 mg 1 qod
Digoxin 0.3 mg q 6–8 h until desired effect achieved
Cardura 1 mg bid

BP runs high, suffered mild heart attack about 1 year ago. Patient states that she "has been feeling poorly last few days and is short of breath on excursion." No known drug allergies (NKDA).

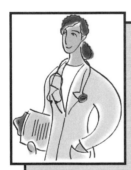

Make a Difference

A patient who presents to your office with chest pain is to be taken seriously. Always document the signs and symptoms and determine if the physician needs to be called immediately. If you are not sure, it is always best to notify the physician of the situation right away. Once you have mastered the skill of determining the rate and rhythm, and basic interpretation of the strip, the need to report to the physician immediately will become apparent.

STANDARD PRECAUTIONS

PPE, ground if applicable

EQUIPMENT/SUPPLIES

Written or verbal order
ECG machine
Electrodes
Conductive gel or gel pads
ECG paper
Mounting device
Examination table
Patient gown (female patient only)
Alcohol or skin cleansing agent
Patient ground (if using older machine)
Disposable razor (male patient)
Mounting paper

STANDARD OF PERFORMANCE OF THE TASK

You may earn a maximum of 5 points for each competency regardless of the number of steps to be performed.

    EX: If you miss two steps and achieve all the rest then you have earned 3 points.

    More than five steps missed means that you have 0 points.

    Your instructor may choose not to assign points but check you off on a pass or fail status. Regardless, you may need to repeat the competency for successful completion.

    It is up to your instructor to determine the maximum number of tries before the competency has been met successfully in the time allotted.

Student Name: _____   Date: _____

Time: Satisfactory   Unsatisfactory

Successful Completion: Yes   No

Grade/Points: _____   Pass   Fail

Need to Repeat: _____   Number of Attempts: 1   2   3

Instructor Comments: _____

_____

_____

CONDITIONS UNDER WHICH THE STUDENT IS EXPECTED TO PERFORM THE TASK

Follow Task/Performance Steps

	Task/Performance Step	S	U
1.	Student gathers equipment and supplies, prepares room for patient, and performs aseptic hand washing. *Gathering supplies in advance assists with organization and time management. Hand washing prevents cross-contamination.*		
2.	Student warms conductive gel as applicable or prepares the electrodes. *Warming gel maintains comfort for the patient and prevents cold gel from touching skin, which can affect the quality of the strip.*		
3.	Student greets and identifies the patient. Introduces self and explains the procedure. *Identifying and confirming patient ensures test is performed on correct patient.*		
4.	Student verifies written or verbal order and compares to patient name and patient record.		
5.	Student explains procedure to patient and importance of patient's role in procedure to obtain a quality strip for physician interpretation. Patient states having chest pain and nausea. Student takes vitals. Student determines need for reporting to physician. *Artifacts can appear on the strip, so be sure to explain to patient the importance of remaining still during the procedure, removing all jewelry, emptying all pockets, and removing any metal that may be on clothing (e.g., belt buckle).*		
6.	Student instructs patient to remove upper portion of clothing, explains where to put clothing, to put on half gown (females) with opening in the front and to have a seat on the examination table. State to patient you will return in a few minutes allowing the patient privacy for changing. *Be sure to identify patients who may need assistance and offer assistance with changing and positioning on examination table. In the event of suspecting a real heart attack you would not leave the room.*		
7.	Student knocks on examination room door and identifies self before entering patient room. *You must maintain patient privacy and dignity at all times.*		
8.	Student checks to make sure patient gown is on correctly and all jewelry and metal objects have been removed.		
9.	Student notes any special instructions from the physician. *Some tests require exercise before test to record changes in physical stress.*		

10. Student assists patient in a supine position using pillows as needed for comfort, and preps the skin if applicable. *Some patients have excess hair and may require shaving while others may need abrading due to oily or dry skin. Electrodes must stick to skin with complete contact to ensure a quality strip for interpretation.*		
11. Student ensures arms are placed flat on the examination table at the patient's side and instructs patient to breathe normally.		
12. Student provides a drape as needed for privacy and patient comfort.		
13. Student records patient's database information, including vital signs and current medications, and notes date and time.		
14. Student checks the machine for safety and grounding positioning the power cord away from the patient.		
15. Student turns on the machine to warm stylus, warms hands, and places gel electrodes or contact electrodes on skin to the chest and limbs appropriately. *If using electrode cups for chest leads, apply a small amount of conductive gel, compress bulb to create suction, press it against the patient's chest at first position, V1, and release bulb and follow the same procedure for the remaining chest leads.*		
16. Student attaches chest and limb leads to electrodes appropriately. *The limb leads are labeled RA, LA, LL, RL, and chest or precordial leads are V1–V6. Some leads are color coded.*		
17. Student checks for accuracy of lead placement, ensures there are no tangles, and leads are contour to patient's body. *It is not necessary to touch the patient's body as you bend with your body to hook up the electrodes. Respect their dignity and personal space when you can. There is no need for any body section to remain uncovered during the procedure.*		
18. Student centers the stylus if applicable, presses the standardization button, and sets on RUN 25. Current machines will perform this function automatically. Follow manufacturer recommendations for the type of machine you are using or follow your instructor's suggestions. *The mark should be 2x10 mm or two small squares wide by ten small squares high. Adjust if necessary. This is also a good time to check for artifacts.*		
19. Student informs patient the test will begin and to breathe normally.		
20. Student begins running the strip. *This is a good time to check for leads not properly attached because it will be apparent at this time.*		
21. Student obtains a readable strip of leads I,II, III and proceeds manually to aVR, aVR, and aVF.		
22. Student obtains a readable strip of leads V1–V6 for 6–8 in of paper. If your machine does not progress automatically you will need to mark your leads at this time. *Some machines do not progress automatically, so you will need to move your chest leads manually to the next position. Be sure to turn the machine off and restandardize each time.*		
23. Student completes test, turns off machine, and informs patient test is complete and to relax. *Do not remove electrodes and leads until physician has viewed the strip and has determined it is a quality strip for interpretation.*		
24. Student removes leads and electrodes and any conductive gel, removes equipment from patient area while ensuring patient privacy.		
25. Student instructs patient to dress, where to dispose of dirty patient gown, and explains the physician will be in to speak with them. Leaves room and allows for privacy.		

26. Student ensures patient name and any pertinent information is on the strip. Most machines will automatically perform this function because you entered the information before starting the test.		
27. Student determines rate and rhythm. If your machine automatically provides you with this information calculate the rate and rhythm to see how accurate you are.		
28. Student unrolls strip and identifies the area to be mounted, starting with the standardization mark. Cut all strips according to the length of the mount or protocol of physician. Repeat until all leads have been mounted. This step may be optional with your instructor. *Be sure all mounts are labeled correctly with patient name.*		
29. Student returns to patient room, knocking before entering, asks if patient has any questions and clarifies.		
30. Student thanks patient, gives any appropriate instructions, making sure there are no further questions.		
31. Student cleans equipment appropriately, disinfects area, and washes hands.		
32. Student documents. • Student had identified the need for reporting the chest pain to the physician before starting the ECG. The physician determined there was nothing serious and allowed the patient to leave with instructions of a follow-up visit in 1 week or to call the office if the symptoms are persistent. • The physician thanked the assistant for bringing the patient's condition to his attention.		

Key: Satisfactory = S; Unsatisfactory = U

Your instructor will review your strip or mounted strip for accuracy and quality. Staple your strip to this page mounted or unmounted.

PROGRESS NOTE – DOCUMENTATION

Name Student/Patient _____

DOB _____

Allergies _____

Gender _____

Date _____

Rate _____   Rhythm _____

_____

_____

_____

_____

Current Medications _____

_____

_____

Practicum 41. Respiratory Testing

COMPETENCY

CAAHEP: 3. b. (3) (b) Perform respiratory testing
ABHES: 4. (ee) Perform respiratory testing

SPECIFIC TASK

This competency may vary depending on the equipment available in your laboratory. Your instructor may choose to have you perform a different type of respiratory testing. Follow the manufacturer's step-by-step instructions to achieve competency. Role-play the scenario below.

Role-play using a classmate as the patient. A patient presents to your office that is asthmatic and is in respiratory distress. Student is able to identify symptoms of respiratory distress, monitor oxygen saturation, and report findings to physician. Student initiates treatment as ordered by the physician. Student instructs patient on use of Peak Flow Meter to be used at home to monitor respiratory condition.

STANDARD PRECAUTIONS

PPE, soap, water, and disinfectant

EQUIPMENT/SUPPLIES

Pulse oximeter
Attached physician orders
Oxygen tank/oxygen facemask or nasal cannula with tubing
Medication (inhaler)
Peak flow meter
Attached daily record chart for peak flow monitoring

STANDARD OF PERFORMANCE OF THE TASK

You may earn a maximum of 5 points for each competency regardless of the number of steps to be performed.

EX: If you miss two steps and achieve all the rest then you have earned 3 points.
More than five steps missed means that you have 0 points.
Your instructor may choose not to assign points but check you off on a pass or fail status.
Regardless, you may need to repeat the competency for successful completion.

It is up to your instructor to determine the maximum number of tries before the competency has been met successfully in the time allotted.

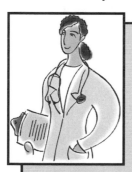

Make a Difference

There are too many deaths despite current treatments for control and reducing asthma-related attacks. Good assessment skills, quick intervention, and patient education are the key to reducing the number of patient deaths!

Student Name: _____   Date: _____

Time:	Satisfactory	Unsatisfactory
Successful Completion:	Yes	No
Grade/Points: _____	Pass	Fail
Need to Repeat: _____	Number of Attempts: 1 2 3	

Instructor Comments: _____

_____

_____

CONDITIONS UNDER WHICH THE STUDENT IS EXPECTED TO PERFORM THE TASK

Follow Task/Performance Steps

Task/Performance Step	S	U
1. Student gathers supplies, performs aseptic hand washing, and applies PPE. *Although asthma is not considered contagious, many respiratory diseases are. It is always good practice to wear a mask until you know the patient's condition.*		
2. Student identifies patient in respiratory distress, assesses for distress symptoms, and states symptoms to physician (instructor). *Good respiratory assessment skills will assist the physician in determining which tests and treatments will benefit the patient.*		
3. Student applies pulse oximeter to patient's left or right index finger quickly and appropriately, identifies patient pulse rate and oxygen saturation. Student assesses the patient's vital signs. *Pulse oximetry is a quick, noninvasive way to determine how well the patient is oxygenating the tissues. Saturation should be at 95 or above.*		
4. Student notifies physician (instructor) of patient in distress and assessment findings of a pulse ox of 82. *A patient identified in respiratory distress requires the physician's immediate attention. Don't forget there are positions such as Fowler's or Semi-Fowler's that will help the patient breathe easier.*		
5. Student obtains verbal/written physician orders, explains to patient plan of care, and carries out treatment as ordered by physician. *If medical assistant has any questions regarding physician's orders, be sure to clarify with physician to prevent medical error.*		
6. Student begins to carry out orders by attaching tubing to oxygen tank and mask or nasal cannula. Open oxygen tank and place mask/cannula on patient's face and set oxygen flow per liter as ordered by physician. *Young children and confused or incoherent patients may need oxygen mask held close to the face.*		
7. Student obtains medication (inhaler) as ordered by physician. Asks questions regarding patient allergies, and instructs patient on the use and inhalation of medication. Temporarily remove O_2 to administer Ventolin. See written orders.		
8. Student continues to monitor patient's respiratory effort, symptoms, vital signs, and O_2 saturation for improvement. *If patient does not improve with current treatment, more aggressive treatment may be required. Notify physician if no improvement or patient becomes worse.*		

9. Student assesses for improved respiratory condition with more effective respirations and increased oxygen saturation.		
10. Student notifies physician of patient improvement and receives order to wean oxygen. *Weaning oxygen (lowering concentration of oxygen) allows gradual assessment of respiratory condition and oxygen concentration, with goal to remove oxygen as tolerated by patient.*		
11. Student weans oxygen, continuously monitors patient, and removes oxygen as tolerated by patient.		
12. Student notes marked improvement with assessment skills and patient feedback.		
13. Student informs physician of patient improvement and receives order to educate patient on home use of peak flow meter to monitor respiratory condition. *Peak flow meter testing is used for patients to identify respiratory condition and level of intervention needed, which gives direction to the patient for treatment.*		
14. Student sets the perimeters for the three-zone management system as follows: Green/580, Yellow/465, Red/290 and states to instructor actions to be taken for each. *Be sure to follow the physician instructions or the zone reference chart for setting perimeters.*		
15. Student instructs patient that the red indicator must beat the bottom of the scale for accurate results. *QC and accuracy*		
16. Student instructs patient to hold peak flow meter upright being careful fingers do not block opening in the back of the meter.		
17. Student instructs patient to stand upright and inhale deeply, placing mouth around mouthpiece creating a tight seal.		
18. Student instructs patient to blow out as hard and fast as possible. *This causes the indicator to move up the scale. The final position is the peak flow rate.*		
19. Student instructs the patient to repeat steps 15 and 18 two more times for a total of three attempts.		
20. Student takes the highest reading and records with the date and time in the daily record chart.		
21. Student instructs patient on documenting peak flow results at home in the daily record chart. *Using the daily record chart gives vital information to the physician for asthma control and effective treatment plan for the patient.*		
22. Student reviews and gives patient peak flow meter instructional brochure with peak flow meter to take home.		
23. Student explains care and cleaning of meter as directed in brochure.		
24. Student allows for patient questions and clarification.		
25. Student thanks patient, cleans area, and washes hands.		
26. Student documents testing, results, O_2 procedure, and patient education in patient record.		

Key: Satisfactory = S; Unsatisfactory = U

PHYSICIAN'S ORDERS

Dr. Franklin Pierce Wright, Family Practice
2310 Wright Way
Melbourne, FL 32904
Telephone (904) 565-3200

Patient: _____

Date of birth (DOB): _____

2 L O_2/min via face mask

   Ventolin Inhaler-2 puffs stat.

  Wean O_2 as pt. tolerates

Instruct patient on use of peak flow meter   Dr. Wright

DAILY RECORD CHART

Patient Name _____

Time	Date								
850									
800									
750									
700									
650									
600									
550									
500									
450									
400									
350									
300									
250									
200									
150									
100									

PROGRESS NOTE – DOCUMENTATION

Name Student/Patient _____

DOB _____

Allergies _____

Date _____

_____

T _____   BP _____   P _____   R _____

_____

_____

_____

_____

SMART THINKING

The following will help you with spelling of medical terms and understanding the definitions.

1. Name at least 4 respiratory diseases/conditions.

1. _____

2. _____

3. _____

4. _____

2. Name at least 6 abnormal respiratory patterns.

1. _____

2. _____

3. _____

4. _____

5. _____

6. _____

Practicum 42. CPR and First Aid

COMPETENCY

CAAHEP: Mandatory - Provider level CPR certification and first aid training
ABHES: 4. (e) Recognize emergencies
          4. (f) Perform first aid and CPR

SPECIFIC TASK

1. **Emergency…emergency!** In the time specified by your instructor, manage a wound that will not stop bleeding using all basic first aid training and OSHA guidelines if applicable.

   Scenario: Role-play with a classmate. You walk into the classroom/laboratory to find a fellow classmate lying on the floor bleeding profusely from the left lateral knee. In spite of your first aid measures, the bleeding will not stop. Role-play and call your area emergency help line for assistance. Continue to apply pressure until the team arrives.

2. Perform CPR in the time specified by your instructor using a mannequin. You may follow the steps outlined in a provider level manual or use the steps below. Once you have successfully achieved certification or if you have achieved certification using a source outside your class, attach a copy of your card below. Your certification must be current.

3. Follow the instructions and implement an emergency plan for your office.

STANDARD PRECAUTIONS

PPE, soap and water, biohazard container

EQUIPMENT/SUPPLIES

Mouth shield or a piece of plastic with a hole for the mouth, clean or sterile. First aid supplies applicable for applying pressure to a bleeding wound. Supplies may vary.

STANDARD OF PERFORMANCE OF THE TASK

You may earn a maximum of 5 points for each competency regardless of the number of steps to be performed.

   EX: If you miss two steps and achieve all the rest then you have earned 3 points.

   More than five steps missed means that you have 0 points.

   Your instructor may choose not to assign points but check you off on a pass or fail status.
Regardless, you may need to repeat the competency for successful completion.

   It is up to your instructor to determine the maximum number of tries before the competency has been met successfully in the time allotted.

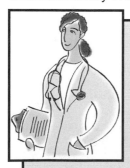

Make a Difference

Learning CPR, first aid, and responding to emergencies are critical concepts that you will use in your profession daily. Learning to recognize heart attack, stroke, cardiac arrest, or foreign-body airway obstruction (FBAO) through instruction and certification will benefit you, the patients you serve, and your family and friends. You will become a valuable member of society with these skills. Any victim of an emergency situation can be saved now because you will possess a skill that is greater than gold!

Student Name: _____   Date: _____

Time: Satisfactory   Unsatisfactory

Successful Completion: Yes   No

Grade/Points: _____   Pass   Fail

Need to Repeat: _____   Number of Attempts: 1   2   3

Instructor Comments: _____

_____

_____

CONDITIONS UNDER WHICH THE STUDENT IS EXPECTED TO PERFORM THE TASK

Follow Task/Performance Steps

Task/Performance Step	S	U
STOP BLEEDING		
1. If you have time, wash your hands and put on the examination gloves, face protection, and a gown to protect yourself from splatters, splashes, and sprays.		
2. Using a clean or sterile dressing, apply direct pressure over the wound.		
3. If blood soaks through the dressing, do not remove it. Apply an additional dressing over the original one.		
4. Elevate the body part that is bleeding. You realize in spite of your best effort that you are not able to control the bleeding and you should call emergency medical services (EMS). Ask for assistance in placing the call while you continue to hold pressure over the bleeding wound. *If direct pressure and elevation do not stop the bleeding, apply pressure over the nearest pressure point between the bleeding and heart.*		
5. When the EMT or emergency team arrives, assist as requested.		
6. After the patient has been transferred to a hospital, properly dispose of contaminated materials.		
7. Remove the gloves and wash hands.		
CPR		
1. Shake the patient and ask, "Are you OK?" If there is no response, call the EMS system, or ask someone to call.		
2. Wash your hands and put on examination gloves if possible.		
3. If the patient is not on his/her back, roll the whole body over.		
4. Open the patient's airway by lifting the chin gently upwards with one hand, while pushing downward on the forehead with the other hand.		
5. Place your ear close to the patient's mouth and keep your eyes on the chest and stomach. Look for chest and abdominal movement. Listen for the sound of air moving. Feel for breath on your cheek. These signs indicate that the patient is breathing.		
6. If you do not see, hear, or feel breathing, begin rescue breathing. Turn the hand you are resting on the patient's forehead so that you can also use it to pinch the nose.		

7.	Place a mouth shield over the patient's mouth, and take a deep breath. Place your mouth on the shield over the patient's mouth, making a seal. Then blow into the mouth. Pause and then blow into the mouth again. Watch to see that the patient's chest rises with each breath.		
8.	If you cannot make a good mouth-to-mouth seal, try mouth-to-nose breathing if needed		
9.	If the patient has a tracheotomy, breathe into the stoma after closing of the mouth and nose.		
10.	Next, locate the carotid pulse to check for a heartbeat. To find the carotid artery, locate the larynx and slide the tips of your index and middle fingers into the groove beside the larynx. If you do not feel a pulse, start artificial circulation.		
11.	Locate the end of the sternum, which is called the xiphoid process. To do this quickly, run your index and middle fingers across the lower margin of the ribs to the notch where they meet. Place the two fingers flat on the chest at this spot. Place the heel of your other hand on the midline of the sternum, next to the index finger.		
12.	With the heel of your hand in position, place your other hand on top of it and interface your fingers. Straighten your arms and lock your elbows. Position your shoulders directly over your hands so that your thrust is downward.		
13.	Depress the sternum 1.5 to 2 inches for an adult. Release the compression completely, but keep your elbows locked and your hands on the chest.		
14.	Do four sets of 15 compressions and two breaths over a 1-minute period. Five compressions and one breath for a 1-minute period if it is a two-person rescue. Then check the pulse.		
15.	If the patient has a pulse but is not breathing, start rescue breathing. If the patient has no pulse and is not breathing, continue CPR until the patient regains consciousness or help arrives. Stop and take a pulse every few minutes.		
16.	Assist EMS personnel as requested. Dispose of any material in the appropriate containers. Remove the gloves and wash your hands.		

Key: Satisfactory = S; Unsatisfactory = U

Attach CPR certification to this page:

3. REMEMBER "PRACTICE MAKES PERFECT"

Every facility should have a "plan of action" when emergencies in the office arise. A good practitioner who works in the front or back office will know what their role is. Everyone should know his/her responsibility, how to activate EMS, and where emergency supplies are kept.

Role-play with four other classmates as though you are the staff below. Have a staff meeting and determine how you will manage one of the scenarios.

On this sheet of paper, prepare a plan for providing for emergencies in an ambulatory care setting, including phone numbers, location of equipment and supplies, and roles and responsibilities of employed health care providers. Use current information from your community.

Creatively think of where and how a plan like this would be implemented. Using triage algorithms is the best way to prepare a plan such as this.

Scenario

Staff: 3 clinical medical assistants, 1 front office medical assistant, and 1 physician
Equipment: Your facility has all required equipment for emergencies.

You may choose either of the following emergencies:

1. 64-year-old man presents to the front office with chest pain.
2. 8-year-old girl presents with snake bite, type of snake unknown, left ankle swollen, bleeding, becoming necrotic.

Plan

_____

_____

_____

_____

Roles/Responsibility

MA #1: _____

_____

MA #2: _____

_____

MA #3: _____

_____

MA #4: _____

_____

Physician: _____

_____

Equipment/Supplies: _____

_____

Location Kept: _____

_____

Emergency #s: _____

_____

Instructor Corrections: _____

_____

_____

_____

_____

Appendix: Selected Answers

Smart Thinking/General Questions: Answers

ADMINISTRATIVE/GENERAL

Although the answers have been provided for you, the faculties encourage you to seek the answers by research or review of your text material and then verify that you are close to the correct response.

    Your instructor will know if you have copied word for word and are indeed looking for your own interpretation of the question.

    Those who cheat are only cheating the patients in the end!

3C2A, 1B, 5C

Scenario #1

The receptionists have breached patient confidentiality by speaking of the patient's condition when it was not necessary. Patient confidentiality should be maintained at all times. Employees should not be discussing patient information unless it directly relates to the treatment or care involved.

    Have regular staff meetings and discuss issues of confidentiality. Present a HIPAA In-service to ensure that all employees understand the serious nature and consequences that can result from breach of patient confidentiality.

Scenario #2:

Mr. Cramer should have been informed of the call and asked to sign a medical record release form before taking any action with the lawyers. One never knows who is on the other end of the phone.

    This would be a good time to review the patient record and allow the patient to complete any additional HIPAA forms that are needed to ensure the patient's privacy and right to patient confidentiality.

3C2B, 1-A, D, G, I-2-P, G-5 F, 6 E

1. Laws are rules and regulations that safeguard society. Ethics are what a individual believes in or a set of moral values.
2. Administrative, clinical, and general duties as defined by that state's Medical Practice Act. Duties will vary from state to state and from office to office as well as in the same clinic. As an example, in the state of Florida, medical assistants cannot perform IV therapy of any kind. If the medical assistant did so, he/she would be practicing outside their scope of practice.
3. Expulsion, suspension, or censure.
4. Always maintain and protect patient confidentiality, show honesty and integrity in your actions, and be knowledgeable and follow all state and federal laws.
5. Identify the nature of the problem, gather all necessary and additional information, think of alternative solutions, and then implement the action, review, and evaluate.
6. The physician works strictly under the AAMA Code of Ethics. The physician should not ask the employee to perform duties that are not within the scope of practice and both should work together as an advocate for the quality of health care.
7. High ethical and moral conduct, diplomacy, professionalism, initiative and responsibility, empathy, courtesy, inter/intrapersonal skills, good communication skills both verbally and written, good hygiene, respect patient confidentiality, accuracy, honesty, integrity, be a team player, and portray a positive self-image.

CMA and RMA

Show initiative, be a team player, and always be honest.

3C2F, 5-E, G

1. August 21, 1996
2. Reducing administrative cost of health care and privacy issues
3. Unique identifiers

4. December 2000
5. Acknowledgment of Receipt of Notice of Privacy Practices – Consent to the Use and Disclosure of Health Information for Treatment, Payment, or Health care Operations
6. Richard Nixon
7. To ensure a healthy work environment and workplace safety
8. DHHS – Department of Health and Human Services, Yes
9. 2 employees must witness the drug being flushed into toilet or sink. Both employees must document on the controlled substance inventory form. For large quantities, you must contact the DEA for instructions.
10. Research article.

3A1A, 3C4C, 3C1D, 2-E, N-3-C, D

1. Patient name and DOB, pharmacy name and number, medication name, spelling, dosage, route, quantity, and any refills.
2. Patient name and phone number where they are at the time of the call, purpose or nature of the call.
3. Patience and listening. Ask how you can assist and show your sincerity.
4. To determine times when the office is closed or the physician is unavailable to see patients or answer questions.
5. 2:00 PM, 1:00 PM, 12:00 PM, and 2:00 PM

3A1C, 3A1D, 3C2C, 3B, 3I

9	Smith	John	
10	Smith	Lori	
11	Smith	John	T.
1	Cooper	Smith	
5	McBride	Debbie	
8	McDonald	Sally	
6	McBride	Deborah	
7	MacBride	Patty	
2	Jones	Kris	
4	Jones	Petunia	J.
3	Jones	Peter	J., Jr.

CLINICAL/GENERAL

3B1A, 4C

1. Viruses, Bacteria, Protozoa, Metazoa, and Fungi
2. Direct contact occurs from person to person. Indirect contact occurs through a vehicle called a vector
3. Medical asepsis destroys the microorganisms after they leave the body while surgical asepsis destroys the microorganisms before they enter the body

3B4B, 3C2E, 4D, 5B

1. Glass mercury, tympanic, thermoscan, tempadot, geratherm.
2. 98.6, 97.6, 99.6
3. Difficulty breathing
4. 96 – Abnormal

3B4C, 3C1B, 3C1C, 2A, F, I, J, K, L, 4A

HEENT: Head, Ears, Eyes, Nose, and Throat
PERRLA: Pupils Equal, Round and React to Light Accommodation
PEARL: Pupils Equal and Reactive to Light
WNL: Within Normal Limits

3B4E, 3B2E, 2B, G, 4H, K, X

- Braxton Hicks are uterine contractions that occur while pregnant.
- Goodell's sign is softening of the cervix; occurs in early pregnancy
- Chadwick's sign is a sign of early pregnancy. Vaginal, cervical, and vulvular tissues turn a bluish-violet color.
- Primigravida is the first pregnancy.
- Secundigravida is the second pregnancy.
- Nulligravida is having never been pregnant.
- EDC – Estimated Date of Conception
- EDD – Estimated Date of Delivery
- VDRL – Venereal Disease Research Laboratory
- RPR – Rapid Plasma Reagin
- Ectopic pregnancy is when the fertilized ovum implants itself but not in the uterine cavity.
- Endometritis is an infection/inflammation of the endometrium.

3B4H, 4N

Disease	Immunization	Description
Diphtheria	DTaP, Td	Protects against diphtheria
Pertussis		Protects against whooping cough
Tetanus		Prevents lock jaw
Hepatitis B	Hep B	Protects high-risk individuals against Hepatitis B. Always have the post titer drawn to make sure the series is working with your immune system
Measles, Mumps, Rubella (German measles)	MMR	This combination of three protects against all three of these viruses
Haemophilus influenzae or meningitis	Hib	Produces immunity against *Haemophilus influenzae* and helps prevent *Haemophilus influenzae* B meningitis
Pneumococcal disease	PCV-7	Helps to prevent pneumonia
Polio	OPV	Protects against polio virus
Varicella zoster (Chicken pox)	Var	Vaccinated early enough, it will prevent the pox

3B3B, 4EE

1. Name at least 4 respiratory diseases/conditions.

1.   Laryngitis

2.   Pharyngitis

3.   Sinusitis

4.   Rhinitis

5.   Asthma

6.   Bronchitis

7.   Pneumonia

2. Name at least 6 abnormal respiratory patterns.

1. <u>Tachypnea</u>

2. <u>Orthopnea</u>

3. <u>Apnea</u>

4. <u>Kussmaul</u>

5. <u>Hypopnea</u>

6. <u>Bradypnea</u>

7. <u>Cheyne-Stokes</u>

8. <u>Dyspnea</u>

Index